SIMULTANEOUSLY SURVIVING CANCER AND CELINDA

Simultaneously Surviving Cancer and Celinda

SSCC

Randy Lawrence

Library of Congress Control Number:		2012917044
ISBN:	Softcover	978-1-4797-1728-6
	Ebook	978-1-4797-1729-3

To order additional copies of this book, contact:
Xlibris Corporation
1-888-795-4274
www.Xlibris.com
Orders@Xlibris.com
121428

Contents

Introduction

Oh my god, where should I start? The reason I decided to put this experience into words is in hopes of removing the shield that has guarded my heart twenty-four seven. I never really had a reason nor a pressing desire to stop loving anyone in my life. So divorce for me was a devastating blow. Now remember as we take this journey, there are three sides to every story—his, hers, and the truth. This is the truth that I experienced. The following chapter is a minihistory of who I am, how I came to be, and the relationships that attributed to my rainbow personality.

Chapter 1

My Minihistory

Right around six in the evening on Tuesday, September 22, 1953, a speeding green 1953 Chevrolet Bel-Air four-door sedan proceeded down Little Creek Road in Virginia Beach, Virginia, en route to DePaul Hospital, located in Norfolk, Virginia, with Russell Henry Lawrence, the worried father at the wheel, and Melissa Caffee Lawrence, the mother experiencing unbearable pain on the rear seat. Melissa called for Russ Henry, and he replied immediately with "Don't call me, I'm driving!" Just as the zooming Chevy began to enter the demarcation that separates the adjacent cities, the corpulent lady produced a nine-pound baby boy, who was given the name of Randy Bernard Lawrence.

After a couple of days at the hospital, I returned home with my mother and father for an informal introduction to my siblings, Wilbert Henry (nine years old), Olivia Estelle (eight years old), Barbara Sue (six years old), Russell Page (four years old), and Patsy Michelle (one year old). They all marveled at such a gross, ugly-looking baby. Daddy was a farmer and Mama was a housewife caring for six rambunctious children. Living on a farm was quite an adventure, with animals galore and numerous jobs to keep my other brothers and sisters busy. Mama definitely needed that for she was pregnant again, and the family once again was exceedingly excited about the future occurrence. On June 24, 1955, we welcomed not one but two additions to the family. What a surprise! Daddy and Mama once again returned home with Mattie and Frances, our new twin baby girls, and what doll babies.

With the family expanding tremendously, Daddy found it necessary to obtain a second job. On the first quarter of the year, he joined the Princess Anne County Police Department, now known as the Virginia Beach Police Department. In March 1957, Mama became pregnant again, which was a blessing. It was September 22, 1957, and what a day! It was my parents' wedding anniversary, Mama's birthday, and my birthday. Mama prepared a gustatory birthday cake with four blue candles while waiting for Daddy to return with her wonderful surprise. Suddenly, Mama was stricken with excruciating pains in her abdominal area. She was taken to bed, and Mama Dizzier, my parental great-grandmother, arrived to administer first aid. Daddy soon returned home and immediately rushed Mama to the hospital. However, it was too late because Mama was hemorrhaging and died shortly after being admitted. It was a very sad and emotionally draining day. I was too young to grasp what was really happening; however, my mother's beautiful, peaceful face is forever logged in my memory. She was dressed in pink and lying asleep in a pink casket as I viewed from the arms of my Uncle Thedo, Mama's youngest brother. The talk of the town was "Lord, what in the world is Russ Henry going to do with those eight children." Well, we were split up and living with all kinds of relatives. That did not last for long; Daddy was determined to raise all of his kids under one roof. One year and three months after Mama's dolorous departure, Daddy remarried an older beautiful and sophisticated lady named Alice Petty. Daddy strongly encouraged us to call her Mama, which we all did as his obedient children. Along with the new stepmother came a stepbrother, John Anthony Petty (JA), and five rooms were added to our home. JA was between Barbara Sue and Page age wise. Hence, the bedrooms were paired in the following manner: Daddy and Mrs. Alice, Henry and JA, Olivia and Barbara Sue, Page and I, and Patsy, Mattie, and Frances, making a huge sleeping quarters for one big happy home. We're just one big happy family, although I spent so many times crying alone and wanting Mama to come back.

Let me take a moment to tell you about Daddy. Daddy was the greatest man in the world to me. He was the strongest, most intelligent, and handsomest man in our neighborhood. Practically all the ladies wanted him, and most were verbal with their desires. Daddy feared no man, but throw a dead man in the same room with him and he would have probably killed himself trying to escape. Daddy was a strict disciplinarian who hits first then asks questions later, and I feared him to no end.

Summers were always a great time for me because we get to spend it at Mama Sue's house, my maternal grandmother. She lived in Nimmos, and three of Mama's siblings and her sister, Aunt Alice, shared her home, which is about fifteen miles away from Creeds where we resided. My Aunt Bertha, Uncle Clay, and Uncle Thedo would each take a week off and take us to the beach and plan some great activities that kept us occupied throughout our summer visit. There was never a dull moment at Mama Sue's house. Unfortunately, that all came to an abrupt halt when my Uncle Clay accidentally shot his pregnant wife, Mary Ruth, and she did not survive. Mrs. Alice not only cut out the summer visits but also minimized the communication between us and Mama Sue, which amounted to almost zero. Boy did I go through emotionally draining withdrawal moments, for Mama Sue just had an unconditional way of making me feel so special.

Every October, during my adolescent years, my Uncle Shelton (his nickname was Tucker), who married my Daddy's only sibling, Aunt Naomi, would take my cousin Shelton and I around all the car dealerships to capture a glimpse of all the new cars from the big three: General Motors, Chrysler, and Ford motor companies. Shelton and I would collect the books of all the different models and read them from cover to cover. We knew all the cars inside out and did not mind showboating our expertise. This was the inception of my developed passion and obsession with automobiles, with Chevrolets always being my favorite. Uncle Shelton did a lot with Shelton and always included me in their many expeditions, whether it was horseback riding or just going to the Freedom 7 Drag Strip, I always felt welcome. Uncle Shelton was also responsible for assigning me nicknames such as Brut or Brut Bernard. And once he asked me, "Am I your uncle, or are you my uncle?" Of course, I said that I was his uncle and called me uncle for years.

Grammar school was fascinating. What a wonderful feeling to see so many little people congregate in one building. A few experiences during elementary school will probably always stay in my memory. One of them was when I was in the second grade in Mrs. Lewis's class. Mrs. Lewis stepped out of the class for a few minutes and left Ann Creekmore in charge. The moment she exited the classroom, Vincent Etheridge jumped on the top of his desk, zipped down his pants, and exposed his penis with one handing holding it and the other pointing at the females while shouting, "Hey, girls! You see this? Every one of you in this class is going to get this!" In a flash, he was all zipped up and back in his seat as though nothing happened. There was complete silence that moment, and shortly afterward, Mrs. Lewis returned to class. No one even mumbled a word regarding the shocking penis display. Mrs. Lewis went on teaching, and Vincent got away with his instant flashing with narration. When I was in the third grade, I remember sitting in the bus in the school parking lot on a seat behind my first cousin, Shelton, who was eating a peanut butter and jelly sandwich. I was staring at the sandwich because it looked so tasty when Shelton asked if I want a piece. I instantly replied yes, and then he smashed the sandwich all over my face. Also in the third grade, Shelton was going out with Shirley Seltzer, and I had a huge crush on Marguerite Parkers. Back then, Daddy allotted us four cents daily for us to purchase milk to accent our homemade lunch. Anyway, we were in the lunch room and Shelton went over to the table where Shirley and Marguerite were sitting. Shelton told Marguerite that I like her, and she responded, "Shelton, tell Randy that if he wants to go out with me, he needs to buy me some cookies." Shelton relayed the message, and I expeditiously took my four cents, purchased four cookies, and rapidly gave them to Shelton to appease Marguerite's request. Once Marguerite had the cookies in her possession, she said, "Shelton, please tell Randy that I do not want to be his girlfriend anymore." That was my first experience of finding love and losing it in ten minutes. The third grade also brought the assassination of President John F. Kennedy. When the announcement was made over the intercom, the whole class including our teachers started crying. It was like losing a family member. We loved President Kennedy. He was beginning to alleviate the second-class citizen status of the black man.

Then there was the fourth grade when I lost control of my bowels, and before I could get out of classroom, feces where running down my pants and on the floor, making a zigzag pattern trail on the floor down the hallway all the way to the boys' restroom. I was so humiliated; however, Daddy's father, Daddy Russ, came to pick me up from school. Daddy Russ had a special way of making light of a situation with humor, which made the ride home a pleasant but funky one. I remember hearing him say something like, "Randy, I am sure you thought it was going to be a little gas, I bet you were totally surprised when liquids and solids commence shooting from your man hole." I did not think that I would ever be able to face everyone at school again. The next day, I returned to school. I heard kids whispering there is Randy Lawrence, the boy who was dragging dodo down the hallway yesterday. I had to laugh because it was even funny to me by then, thanks to Daddy Russ's sense of humor about the embarrassing moment.

During elementary school, I experienced a second death in the family in November 1964. Daddy's father, Daddy Russ, passed always from lung cancer. It was my first funeral after Mama's, and by then I knew that death was a permanent state because after all of my tears, wishes, prayers, and sadness, Mama did not return. This time, it was an immediate eruption of emotion, and I cried like a baby. The pain was so intense at that moment; I thought that I would never recover from this loss of a vital family member. I remember I was helping Shelton deliver the *Journal and Guide* (a weekly local black newspaper) to some of the teachers at school when we heard the news. Uncle Shelton was waiting for us in the school's parking lot. Shelton and I held up pretty good until we reached the last stop, and there in front of the door of the classroom, we began to cry profusely for a few moments. We slowly regained our composure and made the delivery. Daddy Russ's funeral was one sad event. He was a man that seemed like everyone admired. At the funeral when the pallbearers were carrying out his casket, one of them tripped, and they almost dropped the casket. At that moment, Daddy Russ's sister, Aunt Eva, cried out, "Lord, don't hurt him!" I had to smile on that one myself. It did not ease the pain but gave a few folks a chuckle. However, the pain slowly dissipated with time.

As soon as I was old enough for chores, which occupied my evenings after school, I was responsible for taking out the trash, gathering the eggs from the hen house every morning, letting the cow to graze, slopping the hogs after school, and working in the fields as needed. At the age of twelve years, my father instructed me on driving a tractor, which was a dilemma. After demolishing the rear of Daddy's royal blue 1960 Chevrolet Impala four-door hardtop, plowing into Mom Mattie's front porch, crashing into the gas pump by the barn, and periodic trips to the ditch, I became an expert tractor driver.

I have two more memories I would like to share, and I promise to stop with the stories from elementary school. I was in the sixth grade at the time, and I'm not certain of my actions that resulted in the detention assignment, which meant that recess outdoors was revoked that time. Mrs. Reid, my teacher, has also assigned detention to a student named Johnny Bailey, who had been retained at least a couple of years so he was much bigger than everyone else. It was Johnny Bailey, me, and a couple of other students serving detention in class during recess time with no adult supervision. It was not clear then and I do not understand to this day the reason behind Johnny Bailey slapping me around the classroom. It felt like more than fifty slaps; every time I stop moving from one slap, another one immediately followed in rapid succession. I was so afraid; I literally thought that he was going to slap me to death for no apparent reason.

Then there was the summer between my sixth and seventh grade. I was driving the tractor with a plow attach carrying a couple of bags of soybeans to Mom Mattie's house from the field at McCarroll's place. Shelton was on the tractor with me and juxtaposed standing and leaning up against the left wheel finder. I grabbed the gas lever by the steering wheel to slow the tractor down before making the right turn from the road and into the driveway. Once I turned into the driveway, the tractor took off like a rocket and slammed into the back of our 1960 Impala. I immediately hit the brakes; however, I only applied the right brake pedal, which instantly locked the right rear wheel, and the tractor turned 180 degrees to the right. While still in motion, the plow hit Mom Mattie's front porch, taking out a pillar and half of the porch floor boards, scattering the soybeans everywhere, and knocking the rear light of Patsy's bicycle. It felt like a dream in slow motion, but it happened so fast. When I looked back to digest the damage to the car, the porch, Patsy's bicycle, and the freshly plowed front lawn from the tractor lift's broken left arm, I was devastated. Before I knew it, Daddy was driving up to Mom Mattie's house in his police car dressed in his uniform. He did not say a word; he just kept shaking his head to the left and right at a moderate pace. He looked at me, jumped into the police car, and left the premises like a "bat out of hell" for police duty. I'll never forget the sound of those police car wheels and the smell of burning rubber or the look on Daddy's face when he saw all the damage I had done. That is the one time I did not receive any punishment. To top it all off, when we returned to school in September, Mrs. Reid was also my seventh grade teacher. She gave us an assignment the first day of school to write an essay on what we did during the summer. The next day, when she started going around collecting the papers, she stopped at my desk and asked the reason for me not turning in a paper. I responded with I forgot to write the easy. Then she said in loud voice for all of my classmates to hear, "I guess you have forgotten how you smashed up the rear end of your father's car and tore up and spewed peas on your grandmother's porch with a tractor too?" You could have brought me with a penny after hearing that statement. I thought to myself how in the world did she know about my accident?

That was a permanently scarring moment for me, especially when the class broke out into laughter.

When I was enrolled in high school, Henry, Olivia, Barbara Sue, and JA were attending college. The following year, Page went off to college and left all the livestock and the farming to Daddy and me. Daddy sold all of the livestock, and we stuck to grain farming only. Daddy was promoted to Deputy Sheriff, which changed his schedule, and the workload was left to me. Mrs. Alice left Daddy that year, and they soon divorced. Their divorce puzzled me for the longest because they were always kissing and laughing and always going on dates. I only witnessed one altercation between the two of them in the ten years that they were married. The first episode was when Daddy and Mrs. Alice had taken me shopping to buy an Easter suit in a shop downtown on Granby Street in Norfolk. Once the selection and purchase was finalized, we were about to leave the premises when Daddy handed Mrs. Alice a one hundred dollar bill. She became very irritated and reprimanded Daddy in a hoarse tone pointing out her receiving money from him in the store. Daddy responded with "What would you rather me do, give it to you in the street so someone can knock you in the head and take it away from you?" His statement rapidly ended the argument.

I also remember the night Mrs. Alice left. It was around 7:30 p.m. Patsy, Mattie, Frances, and I were on the couch in the den watching television. Mrs. Alice appeared to be intoxicated and entered the front door asking in a slurred voice, "Is your Daddy here?" We answered no, and she stumbled back to the 1966 Pontiac Bonneville Brougham two-door hardtop and disappeared into the night. We went to bed and, being the sound sleeper that I still am, heard nothing. I was awakened by Mattie and Frances saying, "Randy, Mama's gone!" They told me what they heard. Apparently, Mrs. Alice got home late that night drunk as a skunk, yelling at Daddy about having an affair, and jumped on him on the bed swinging like a sissy. Daddy immediately restrained her on floor and asked Henry to call her sister to apprehend this volatile woman. Mrs. Walk and her husband arrived forty-five minutes later, and they carted her off. That was last time I saw Mrs. Alice, until 1985.

After Mrs. Alice flew the coop, I gained a tremendous amount of weight because the food was no longer rationed in our home. I started eighth grade at Floyd E. Kellam High School and was among the few who dared integration. We had a choice of attending the all-black school Union Kempsville or the high school zoned for our district. All of my five older siblings attended and graduated from Union Kempsville. Patsy had already been attending Kellam for a year. It was quite a transition coming from the all-black Seaboard Elementary School where I knew everyone in school to attending classes where I was a fly in bowl of milk. Between thirteen and fourteen years old, I was six feet one inch tall and weighed a whooping one hundred and ninety-eight pounds, which was distributed in the wrong places (butt and gut). Unfortunately, the teen ache struck around the same time. Some of the kids at school called me fat, black, bumpy face, or bitch. Needless to say, my self-esteem was shot, especially living in the shadow of my handsome brother Page, who was absolutely adored by all girls. In the eighth grade, I got my first real girlfriend, Gwendolyn (Gwen) Holloway. Gwen was black and lovely, with large deep brown eyes, long lean black legs, and extra huge breasts, and she was a sister who wore colorful miniskirts. In addition, she was an amazing singer and a master in the art of piano playing. She did not look like an eighth grader. She wrote me the sweetest love letters, which helped repair some of damage from constant teasing from other students.

I loved high school, with the exception of the verbal abuse I received from some of the older students. I won't mention any last names (two Larry's and a Terrell), but their whole names are forever on the tip of my tongue. They tortured me for two years, calling me a sissy and a punk every opportunity our eyes met and sometimes if they were just in close proximity. Thank god they graduated during the end of my freshman year. I know you are wondering why they would say such a thing. Well, you see when I was young, I did "guy stuff" with the boys in my neighborhood, but I was not so good when it came to sports, so sometimes I would be referred to as a punk. Then I had another interest that involved playing with dolls especially styling their hair, which was an activity I enjoyed with my sisters. I was OK with the term sissy and punk in elementary school because I thought a sissy was a guy who played with dolls and a punk was a guy not athletically inclined. Well, needless to say, sissy/punk had whole new connotation in high school, and I was certainly not meeting those criteria. Life got better during my sophomore year. I was a member of the Library Club. During my junior year, I was vice president. Sophomore was a tragic time for me; I lost someone I admired and held in the highest respect. Dr. Martin Luther King's assignation was devastating and left a tremendous void in my soul. We stayed home from school the day of his funeral, and we heard that the black students that attended on that day were harassed at school. There was even a sign put in the hallway saying "Niggers Go Home."

During my senior year, I was kicked out of the library and placed back in a study hall for dancing in the magazine room with Vanessa Bowser. During my junior and senior years, there was no time for other activities for my after-school hours consisted of farming. After I got my driver's license, my relationship with Gwen became hot and heavy. I was also still growing up and out, so by my senior year, I was six feet two inches tall and two hundred and ten pounds, not very athletic, especially in basketball. Lord knows it was hard growing up in a black neighborhood being tall and black with two left hands and two right feet. I was always the last guy picked when it came to choosing teams. During my senior year, I decided to attend college and was accepted in Norfolk State College. My sociology professor named Mrs. Jesse Jones, a garrulous hoyden, fell in love with my available father. At that time, I attended church every Sunday, holding a position as a school teacher, and was a member of the Junior Choir, the Young Men's Chorus, and the Senior Choir. Mrs. Jones was on the board of the Baptist Society. She nominated me for a $25 book scholarship, which I received. Daddy and Mrs. Jones started dating shortly afterward. Upon graduating from Floyd E. Kellam High School in June 1971, Uncle Clay gave me his white 1960 Chevrolet Impala two-door hardtop with a red interior. That summer, Daddy paid my cousin Herald Junior to paint my baby royal blue and patch up the floor boards.

Late August 1971, I started attending Norfolk State College through a school loan cosigned by my father from the Virginia National Bank. I lived with Cut'in (our pronunciation of the word cousin) Florence, Mom Mattie's first cousin and Shelton's parental grandmother. Cut'in Florence lived two blocks from Norfolk State College in a two-story, high-ceiling, four-bedroom house. Shelton and I lived with Cut'in Florence, with me renting a room from her for $5 a week. During the first semester, I embraced meeting and greeting plus having fun and playing games. My grade point average ended up being 1.4 for the first semester. I also met a nice young lady named Sandra Moyer from Greensboro, North Carolina. I nicknamed her Sun Drops. I desired for us to be more than friends, which ended abruptly when Sun Drops said, "I want a man with blue eyes and blond hair." I knew at that moment that I would never fit that bill. We still became the best of friends and spent lot of time together. During the second semester, I majored in Business Administration, following the advice of First Lieutenant Wilbert Henry Lawrence, who also recommended that I enroll into the Army ROTC program. I informed him of the crack in his skull and stated that I would never join the army. During the second semester, Daddy auctioned the farm equipment and leased his land to a local farmer. My 1960 Impala stopped running and was sold during the auction. However, Daddy purchased a white 1961 Plymouth Valiant four-door sedan for seventy-five dollars. We made another visit to Herald Junior's auto body and paint shop, and I was rolling in royal blue once again. I decided to lose weight after a very embarrassing moment with a young lady who I really wanted to develop a relationship with. Her name was Anita Jones, and she could crack her knuckles by moving her fingers just like me. I knew it had to be love for the cracking of knuckles was a match made in heaven. One evening Anita came over to Cut'in Florence's house to study with me. After we finished studying, we moved into the living room and onto couch where things were going pretty good, until I lifted my arm to place it around her shoulders and she screamed, "I—I what's that?" When looked down, my band lawn shirt had come up and my belly was like Jell-O hanging out, shaking. That was a turning point. I did not study with Anita ever again. In February 1972, I started a diet and looked for employment opportunities. On March 31, 1972, I began my first job at the Seashore State Park during my spring break. Once I started earning money, Sun Drops and I purchased twin Iverson ten-speed bicycles, and the first time we went riding, we completed twenty-five miles. That was the day I developed my passion for bicycling. Once summer came, I was employed at the Seashore State Park full time, working the grave yard shift from midnight to 8:00 a.m. cleaning restrooms in the camp ground.

In addition, that summer, Daddy married Mrs. Jesse Jones. We thought that Mrs. Alice was bad, until Mrs. Jones, whom we were instructed to call Mother, flew in on a boom. Man did she clean the house; within two years, my five siblings that were living at home were gone. She immediately converted three of the bedroom into an office, a walk in closet, and a junk room. There was no room at the inn if children planned to stay a spell.

After the summer, I continued to work at the Seashore on weekends while attending college. I also managed to lose fifty pounds, which changed my life immensely. Activities that were once impossible soon became very possible. Unfortunately, my basketball skills were left untouched. I also stopped renting a room from Cut'in Florence's home and moved into the barracks at the Seashore State Park.

Gwen and I had a very emotional break up. She was interested in having children and getting married, whereas my focus was getting a college degree. Shortly after the end of our intimate relationship, my $75 Valiant was suddenly stricken with a terminal disease (transmission lockup) and died. Daddy suggested buying a brand-new automobile. So in October 1973, I purchased a light blue 1973 Chevrolet Nova hatchback with three on the floor. My car payments were $76.33 monthly. A second job was mandatory to cover my financial obligation, so I found employment with the Budget Marketing Service soliciting magazines door to door after classes. One of my funniest encounters soliciting magazines happened when I knocked on a townhouse in Virginia Beach and beautiful blonde answered the door. I went into my memorized script when a little boy, probably about three years old, came down the stairs to see who was at the door. He stop in the middle of the stairs and said in a loud voice, "Mom there's a chocolate boy at the door; I've never seen a chocolate boy before!" and he kept repeating that statement over and over. I started to laugh, I thought it was cute. The lady turned beet red and started to apologize for her son's behavior and eventually closed the door overcome with embarrassment. I did not make that sale. By the way, I had the highest sale record than any of the other teenage workers.

In January 1973, I adjusted my schedule so that all of my classes were in the morning and began working at the Seashore State Park from 4:00 p.m. to midnight, from Wednesday to Sunday in the Contact Station, which involved assigning campsites and out processing campers. Once there was a camper who was irritated about having to wait by standing in line to be processed for a campsite assignment. He stepped in front of everyone and demanded service, and I asked him to get back in line and told him that he would be serviced in the order that he arrive. He started screaming and I closed the window of the Contact Station in his face and did not open it until he left. Someone pointed him to the park superintendent's office. I did not see the irate camper again after that brief encounter. At the end of my shift, Mr. Joly came down with a big smile on his face and said that some camper came to his office screaming, "That goddamn nigger closed the window in my face!" Mr. Joly said that he replied, "If Randy closed the window in your face, then you don't deserve camping in my park so get off the premises immediately before I have the police remove you." Every summer, Mr. George Joly promoted me to shift leader of the midnight to 8:00 a.m. shift because I possessed great skills in knowing the secret to making a commode smile and because of my outstanding customer service skills. I passed on my phenomenal skills to the other eight personnel and stepped into the supervisory world. Being the shift leader gave me the opportunity to drive around in the Ranger truck, giving the appearance of a real park ranger instead of a Johnny mop.

In September 1974, I changed my major to Accounting because I could not seem to capture the content essences of those boring business courses. That year, I joined the National Association of Black Accountant (NABA), and the following year, I was elected vice president of that organization. NABA sponsored a trip to New York for a convention, and you should have seen this country boy in the big city. It was my first time riding the subway.

In February 1975, I met Celinda in the library on the third floor. I was captivated by the magic in her large brown eyes. It was love at first sight for me. After that moment, I could not get her out of my head. I knew then that she was the one for me. However, there are always two sides to a story, and Celinda thought I was strange. The next day, I searched the campus, found the raving beauty, and poured my heart out to her. I finally convinced her to at least go out with me. Our first date concealed my faith, and all of my loving feelings were confirmed.

The following year, I resigned from the Seashore State Park, moved out of the barracks, and rented a room at a boarding house in Norfolk. I began working at the United Virginia Bank as a part-time drive-in teller, which wasn't enough income. On that note, I was hired by the Tidewater Association for Retarded Citizens as a weekend counselor at the Hope House on Granby Street in Norfolk. I was responsible for planning activities and ensuring that the twelve male residences were learning skills to become self-sufficient.

In May 1975, graduation came quickly, but not for me. I still had many more accounting classes to complete. In September 1975, I enrolled in five accounting courses and managed to pass them all with at least a C. In May 1976, graduation time rolled around again; however, history repeated itself. I received a D in Advanced Accounting and in Auditing, which was the second time. What a disappointment to my father and my wicked stepmother. Unfortunately, neither one of the courses were offered in summer school. I deliberated cashing in the chips on this education thing and just calling it wash with college. Then I thought about all the money and time I invested to stop with only two accounting classes left to meet the graduation requirements. I decided to go back and fulfill the requirements no matter how long it would take. Unfortunately, the two classes I needed were not offered until the following school year during the second semester. The time off from school afforded me a great opportunity to seek different employment options that would increase my financial status. The bank gave me full-time employment as a floating teller. That summer, I stopped working at the Hope House and gained employment with the 7-Eleven Corporation as a night shift manager from 11:00 p.m. to 7:00 a.m. I moved out of Norfolk and rented an apartment in Regency Apartments, three miles from the oceanfront. I furnished it with things from Daddy's barn behind the house and brought living room furniture from Cost Plus using the extra pay I earned from 7-Eleven. I worked eighty-eight hours weekly for the entire summer and first semester. I did not attend college the first semester because the two courses I need for graduation were not offered. During the second semester, I terminated my employment with 7-Eleven and returned to college at night. The Hope House accepted me back as a weekend counselor, and all was well again.

Two weeks before graduation in May 1977, I was fired from United Virginia Bank for refusing to work under the conditions following an involuntary transfer to the downtown office right around examination time. A vacation was mandatory for my sanity. The magnificent week I spent at the beach riding my bicycle and girl watching sufficed. I called Daddy and said I may need to come home if I can't get a job within sixty days. The next week, I went to see Mr. Joly at the Seashore State Park, and he informed me that a job was always available for me there. I went back to the Seashore State Park on the condition that I would be seeking employment that will result in a career in my major area of study. Finally, praise the Lord, I met the graduation requirements to receive a bachelor of science in accounting degree from Norfolk State College. May 17, 1977, Sunday, was graduation day, and I picked up Celinda for she was graduating too. The graduation ceremony was in the Scope in downtown, Norfolk. During the ceremony, I looked into the stands and spotted most of my family. I still remember the proud look on Mama Sue's face from far away. Unfortunately, immediately after the graduation ceremony, I was so depressed I left without interacting with any of my family and went back to my apartment and fell asleep. Somehow, that great feeling of aspiring to become something diminished for now I was just another person with a degree. In June 1977, I began seeking different employment. The middle of June 1977, I began working at the Norfolk Adult Activity Center, which was funded by the Tidewater Association for Retarded Citizens. I resigned at the Seashore State Park once again. I was hired as a group leader for eight mentally retarded adults we called clients. The job was sincerely interesting, and I enjoyed it immensely.

In October 1977, the Hope House laid off all weekend help, including me, which manifested into a financial strain on my tight budget. Food disappeared in my apartment rapidly; food was so scarce that even two flies died from starvation. It was definitely time for another part-time job, so I applied to every local department store. What a blessing when Leggett's hired me as a part-time shoe salesman for Christmas help. I had the highest sale rate of the employees in the shoe department, so my employment was extended. During the holidays, Celinda and I took our relationship to whole new level. I was feeling good man.

In January 1978, Celinda and I had a divergence, which resulted in another termination of our relationship. I was promoted to Vocational Technician at the Norfolk Adult Activity Center, which included a $3,200 a year raise. I was responsible for the work production of sixty clients and in training the low-functioning clients. In addition, I was responsible for accessing each client's individual vocational skills. After Celinda cut me off again, I needed a change of climate and developed a wild hair for something exciting out of the city. In March 1978, I enlisted in the army on the delayed entry program. My family was horrified. However, I needed something to ease my roller coaster heart. In April 1978, Celinda returned with the news of being three and half months pregnant and was sad because of her desires to attend medical school. I unloaded my news of my army commitment, got down on my knees, and proposed to Celinda that night. She said that she did not love or like me too much. I told her half of that child she was caring was mine and I had rights just as she did. So she said yes under the condition that we could divorce after the birth of our child. That way, Uncle Sam would finance the medical expenses, and I legally would have my child to raise. We married for all the wrong reasons. Twelve days later, I resigned from both jobs, and Celinda gave her thirty-day notice to the Norfolk General Hospital prior to my entering the army. The mellifluous days we shared together were imponderable, and the essence of our relationship was conceived.

On July 25, 1978, I was off to basic training at Fort Leonard Wood, Missouri. It was hot and loaded with rocks and skunks. Being almost twenty-five years old while attending basic training was not so bad because I rapidly discovered that they were only mind games. In addition, being physically fit was half the battle. I did have a few things that I had to adjust too. The first was at the reception station where I was processed for a week. The commodes in the bathroom of the barracks were lined up with no stalls. Doing the heavy stuff had always been a private moment for me, and the thought of someone watching me in my moments of relief was horrifying. After a couple of days, I was pretty backed up and had to find relief or else explode. It was about 3:00 a.m. and I could not hold it any longer, so I finally sat on one of the exposed toilets and let it rip. No sooner than things started to move, another soldier entered the bathroom. He not only sat right next to me but also fired up a conversation. I felt like jumping off the pot to escape. Unfortunately, I could not stop things in motion and slowly engaged in the conversation only to find that I was freaking out for nothing. I did a lot of singing in the showers and had a singing rap penned to my name. One day, I was singing in formation, which was definitely a no-no. The drill sergeant started screaming at me, "Goddamn it PFC Lawrence, since you can't refrain from singing in formation, take your ass over there and sing to that goddamn pole." I walked over to the telephone pole and started singing at the top of my lungs—I sang to the goddamn pole over and over again. The drill sergeant's face turned beet red, as the other soldiers did everything to keep their composure, when I yelled out and said to the drill sergeant the pole is vibrating. He responded, "Then fuck it then PFC Lawrence!" With that command, I grabbed the pole and started my chant once again and in the line, and it feels so good. This went on for several seconds until the drill sergeant ordered me back in formation with the other soldiers. The only other problem was learning how to fire the M16. I have never fired a weapon until I joined the army. Even though I grew up on a farm where all of the males were great hunters, I just could not get into killing animals. So the first time on the rifle range, I only hit two of forty targets. Believe me when I say that there was a lot of remediation to aid in finally qualifying and graduating without any complications. Then I attended AIT (Advanced Individual Training) at Fort Benjamin Harrison, Indiana, for finance training. I loved every minute of it for the ratio was 7:1 of women to men. On October 15, 1978, we were blessed with a seven-pound, eight-ounce son, who I named Lamarr Scott Lawrence. Since I did not smoke, I broke the tradition of handing out cigars and distributed tootsie pops to my finance class members. Ten days later, I reunited with my wife and new son. Lamarr was a beautiful child. We called him the golden boy because he enriched our lives immensely. He was a sweet baby, and he hardly ever cried. However, he did not smile until he was four months old, and I told Celinda that we could attribute that to her evil ways during her pregnancy.

On November 1, 1978, upon completion of finance school, Fort Campbell Kentucky greeted me with open arms. Celinda and Lamarr joined me a week later. I thought that Celinda was going to get back in her 1973 Chevrolet Monte Carlo and drive back to Virginia when she saw our new living accommodations. It was a tiny blue two-bedroom trailer. In fact, it was so tiny that our green sofa was the width and the doors slid out of the walls, and to gain access to the master bedroom, one would have to go through the bathroom. Lamarr's bedroom was just big enough for his crib and a diaper pail. Celinda and I fixed it up real cozy and had our first wonderful Thanksgiving and Christmas together, along with several friends of mine that did not go home for the holidays. We only lived in that love nest for three months before Celinda found us a three-bedroom house to rent in Clarksville, Tennessee, right down the street from the famous Grandpa's department store. Fort Campbell was a catastrophic experience, but I had a chance to display my talents by entertaining an audience of 2,000 people during "The Week of the Eagles" as a backup singer for a group that the military community theater put together. I had a degree in accounting but was filing records, and that task got old fast. Finally, someone recognized that I had other skills and transferred me to the disbursing section to be a cashier. It was long before I applied for Officer Candidate School (OCS) to help relieve the tension. I was accepted to OCS and left for Fort Benning, Georgia, on November 1, 1979. OCS was a wonderful experience. I got the chance to take my physical fitness to a whole new level and to showcase my talent in singing. I ran with a fast group and called some mean cadets during some pretty mean run. A great moment for me during OCS was when our company mascot, Dud the Water Bug, passed away. Since I was the religious officer of the platoon, I together with the other religious officers was responsible to give Dud a send-off service. The company stood at parade rest while another candidate delivered the eulogy. I rewrote the lyrics to Barbara Streisand's "Memory" and sang it with feelings, and just as I was beginning to reach the climax of the song, a soldier yelled from the formation "Sing it brother!" and I instantly received the validation of my vocal abilities. After that, Dud got a twelve-toilet flush salute and was flushed with the twelfth salute. Celinda, who was five months pregnant, and Lamarr stayed in Clarksville, and an army buddy of mine, Gregory March, stayed with them to help out. However, it was not long before they joined me in Georgia during the Christmas holidays. We packed a U-Haul and moved into a nice two-bedroom townhouse in Columbus, Georgia.

On March 29, 1980, at Martin Army Hospital in Fort Benning, Georgia, Jason Wells Lawrence, a screaming five-pound, fourteen-ounce baby boy, became a part of our happy family. This was truly a remarkable moment for me. I actually got a chance to witness this miracle. At the hospital, Celinda kept saying that it was time, but the doctor was not quiet in agreement. She was adamant and relayed the message to the powers that be. They rushed her into the delivery room; however, before they could move Celinda from the gurney to the delivery table, the doctor yelled, "Lookout here it comes!" With that statement, the movement stopped, and Jason shot out like a cannonball, which required the doctor to make a complete catch to keep him from hitting the floor. He shot out with such force that the umbilical cord snapped. Tears flowed from my eyes as I watched this unforgettable blessing. The tough part was watching the doctor insert is arm into Celinda to remove the placenta since the umbilical code was severed. It looked like he was raking her insides, and believe me when I say Celinda's facial expression was not the most pleasant. Celinda stayed in the hospital for an additional day because she decided to get her tubes tied. We were soon back home, and Celinda's decision to breast-feed Jason made him an even bigger crab. He would scream if anyone touched him besides Celinda, and that little nerd would not sleep unless he had a nipple in his mouth. Janice, Celinda's younger sister, came to help out shortly after Jason was born. She was a real asset in helping Celinda deal with a new born and the eighteen-month-old Lamarr. Lamarr was known for singing in his crib. One evening while we were sitting downstairs shortly after Janice's arrival, we heard in this high pitched voice "Feel me, I want to feel the fire," being repeated over and over again. With a perplexed expression on Janice's face, she asked, "What was that?" Celinda and I laughed and explained that it was our darling Lamarr singing himself to sleep. Janice stayed for a couple of weeks, and after her departure, Jason's nipple habit was still in full force. With the tension building and with this young lad destroying our sleeping arrangement, I told Celinda one of us had to leave our bed and it was not going to be me. Seems like the moment we started Jason on the bottle, he made a 180-degree turn. It was so wonderful to sleep with my wife without the baby. I got to enjoy holding and playing with Jason. However, poor Celinda was depressed because her 36 D cup breasts rapidly returned to their original size. This made life easier for everyone.

From Georgia, we moved to Fort Eustis, Virginia. It was really nice being back home. I'll never forget when we went to visit Celinda's parents to show off our new addition to the family. I wish that you could have seen the expression on Mrs. Scott's face when she first laid her eyes on Jason. Her mouth was open for a few seconds and then a piercing "oh he's so, he's so precious!" It was a grand experience for me to have access to my extended family for my family always had activities going on. Celinda and I also purchased our first home. It was a three-bedroom, one-bath ranch-style home in Newport News. Armed with my Infantry Lieutenant Bars, an M16 fife, my battle dress uniform, and a silicon tape recorder, I aggressively and singlehandedly attacked the Xerox machine, word processor, and pencil sharpeners with the tenacity and ferocity of a pregnant worm. It was wonderful living back in Virginia for we were near home, and boy how I had missed the Atlantic Ocean and especially my family. The Army Training Board was my first duty assignment after my commission. That was a fantastic wild two years of service, from the immersion of family bond renewal to military service. In fact, when my request for an overseas tour was approved, before we departed in July 1982, the Army Training Board gave a farewell lunch at the Whaling Company in Williamsburg, Virginia. Pat Maddin, a civilian employee, made a book of my experiences at Fort Eustis, and it was presented to me at the farewell luncheon on June 30, 1982.

THE MANY FACES OF LT. RANDY B. LAWRENCE

FROM THE FRIENDS OF
ARMY TRAINING BOARD
FORT EUSTIS VIRGINIA

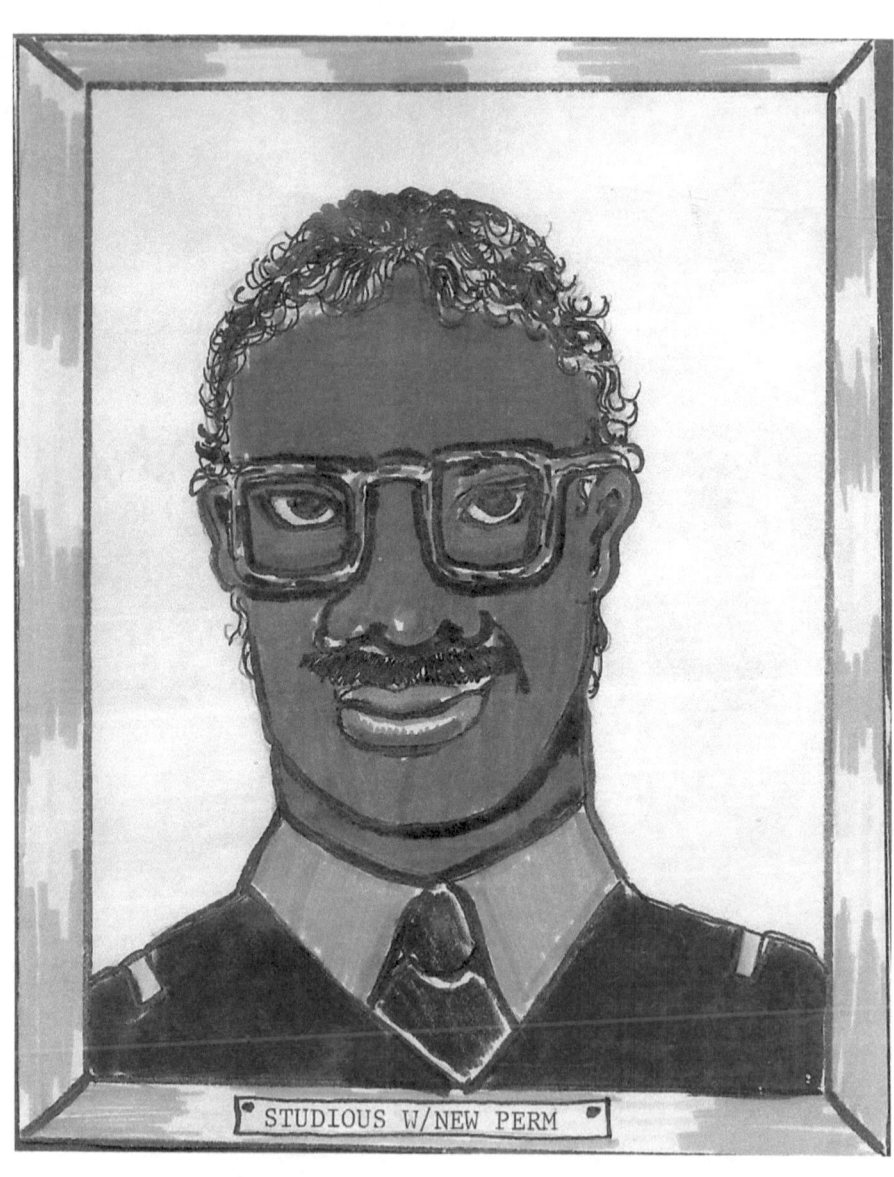

STUDIOUS W/NEW PERM

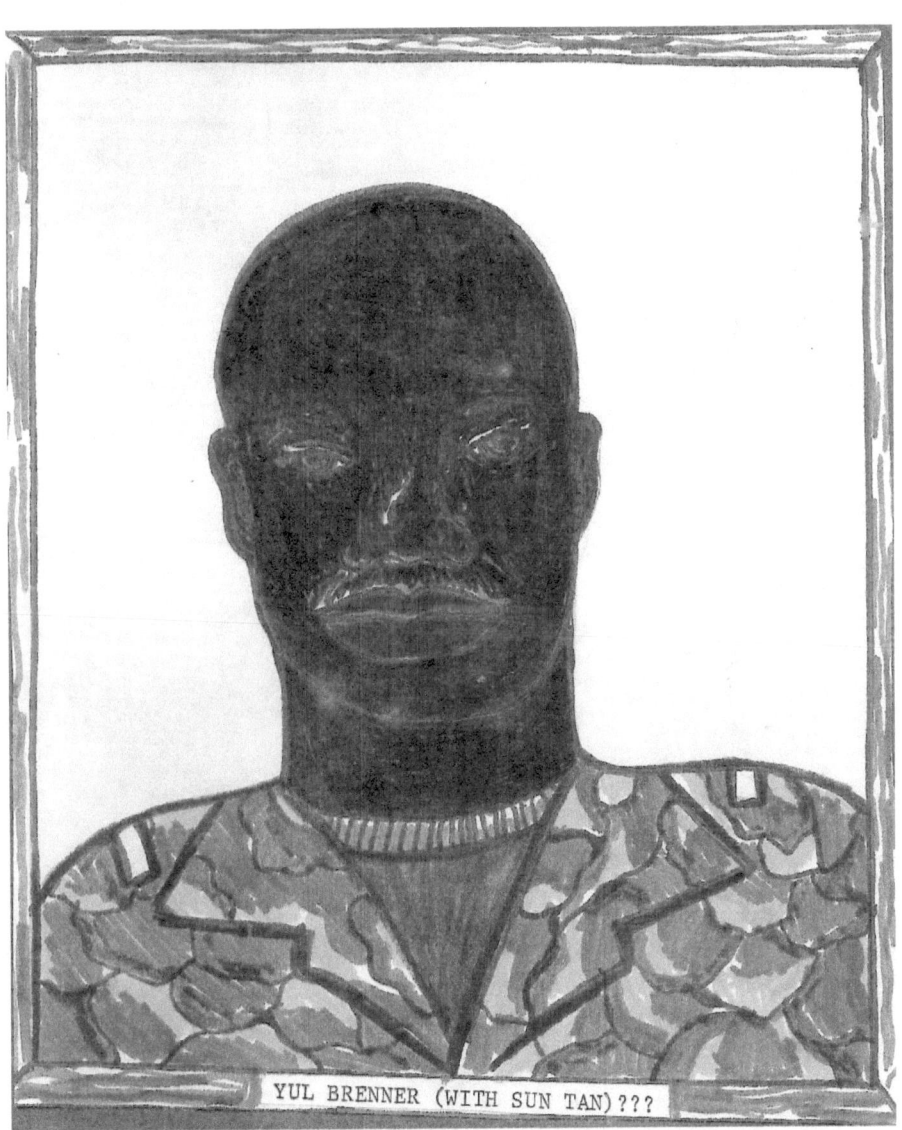

YUL BRENNER (WITH SUN TAN)???

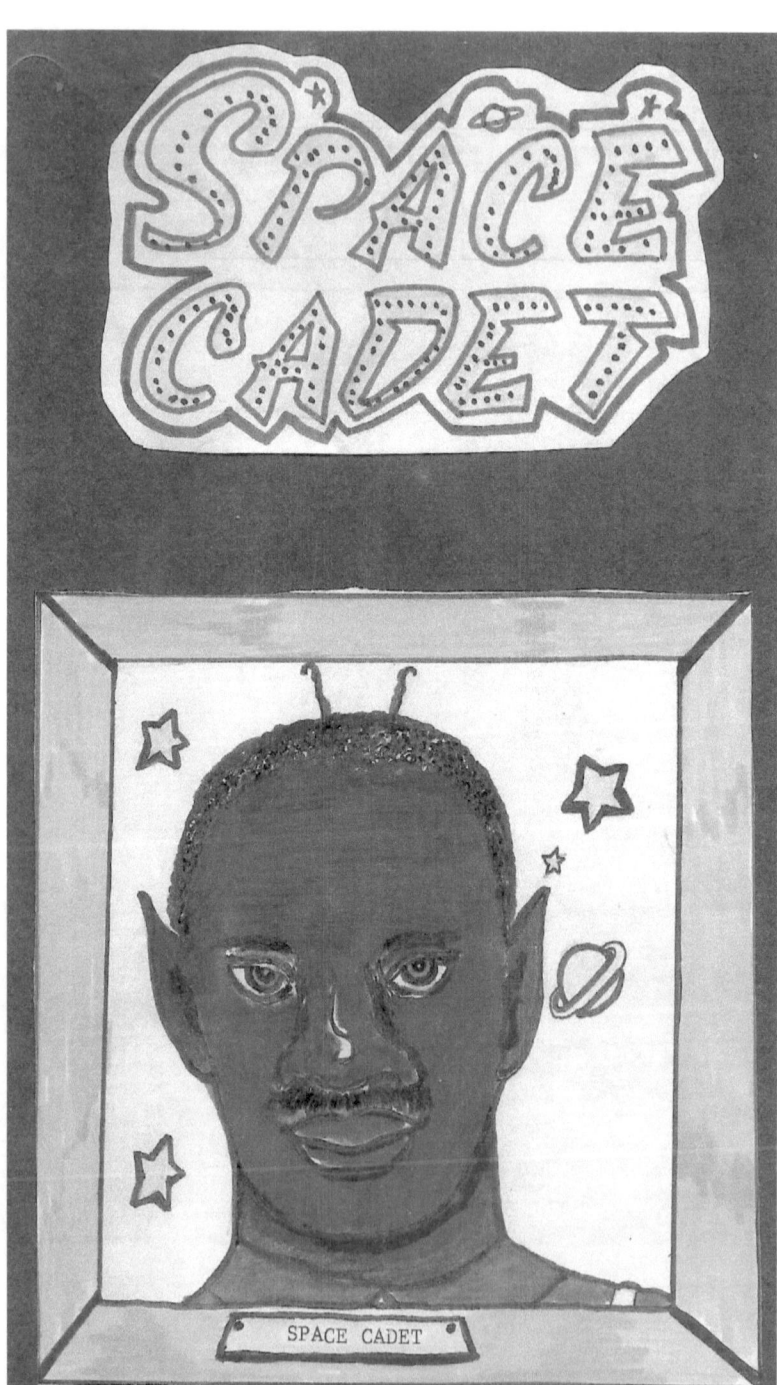

SPACE CADET

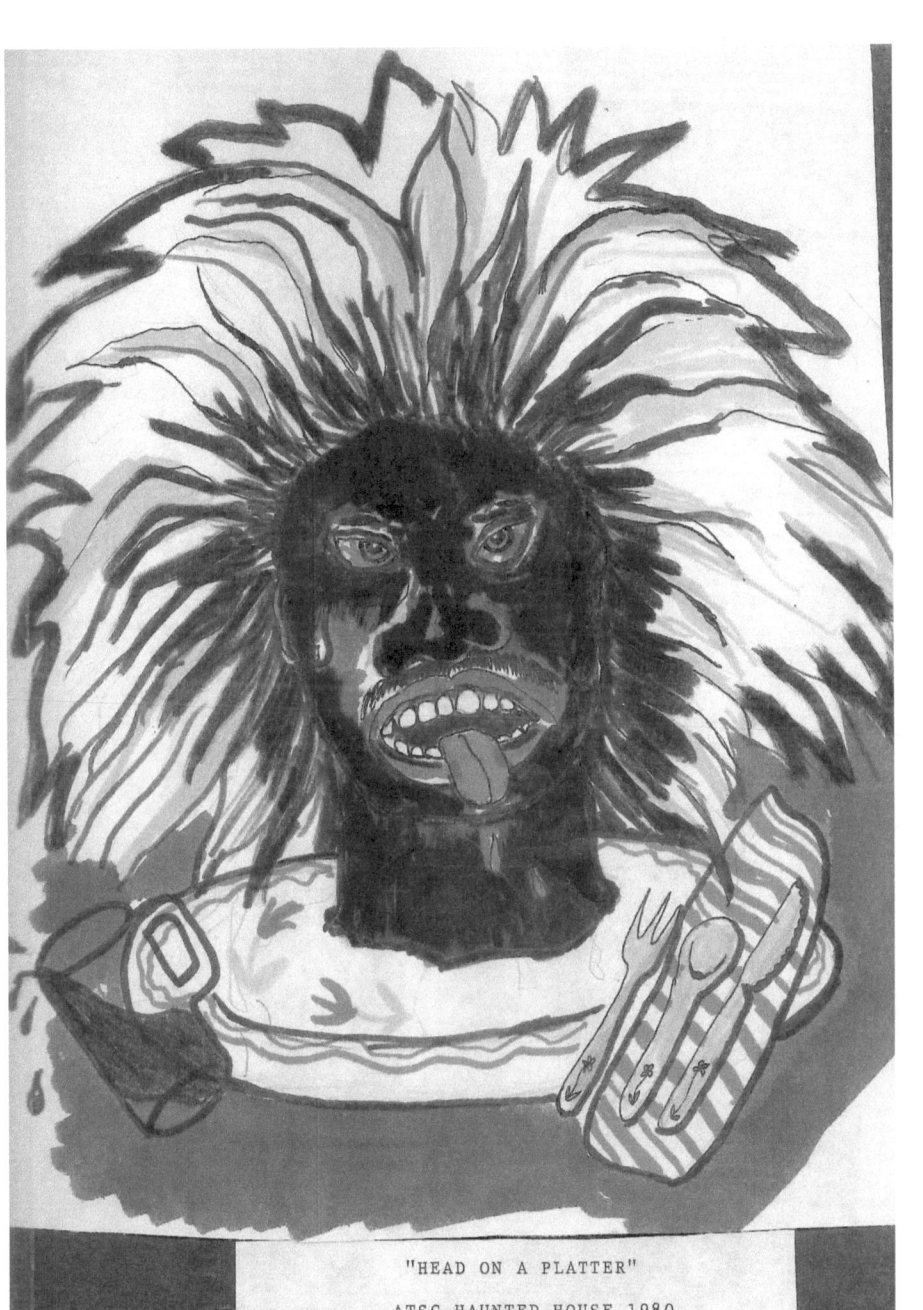

"HEAD ON A PLATTER"

ATSC HAUNTED HOUSE 1980

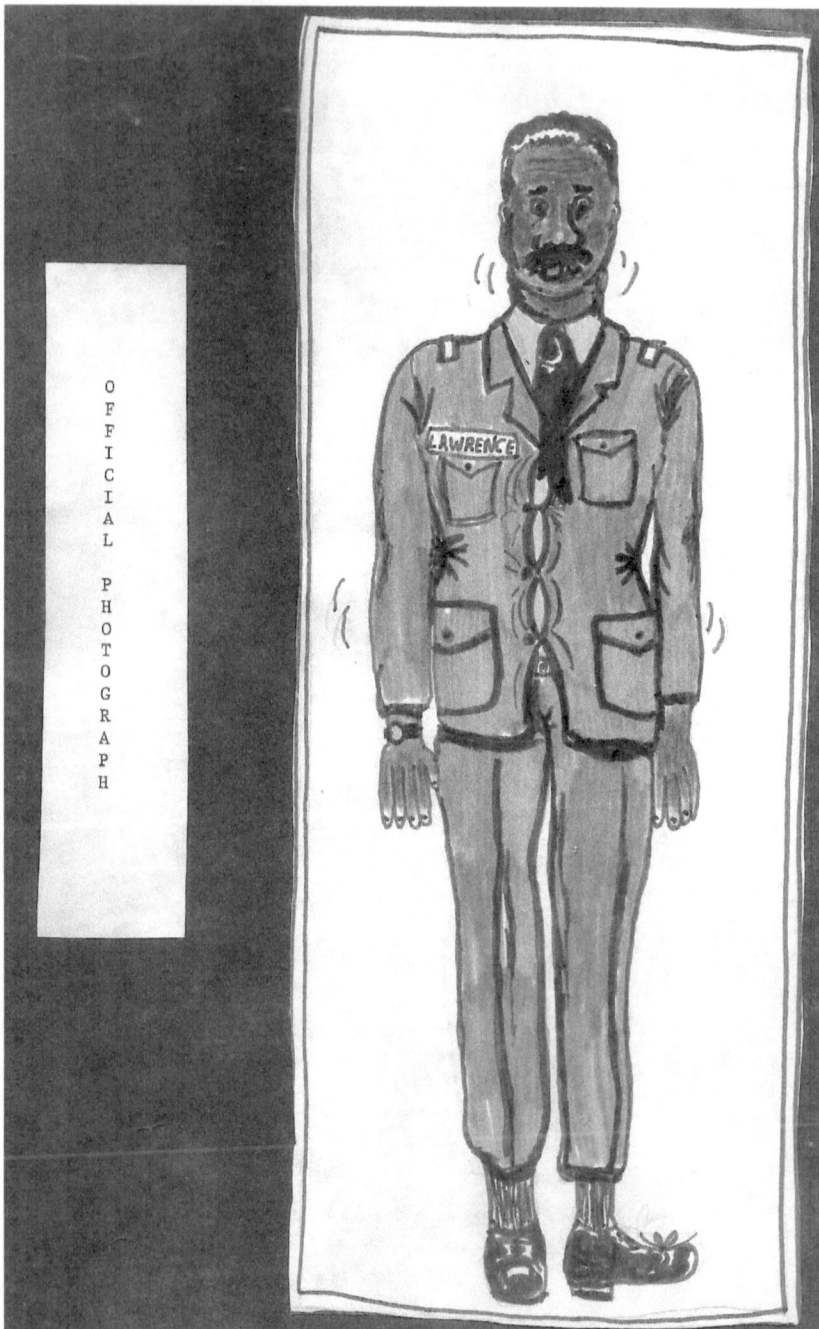

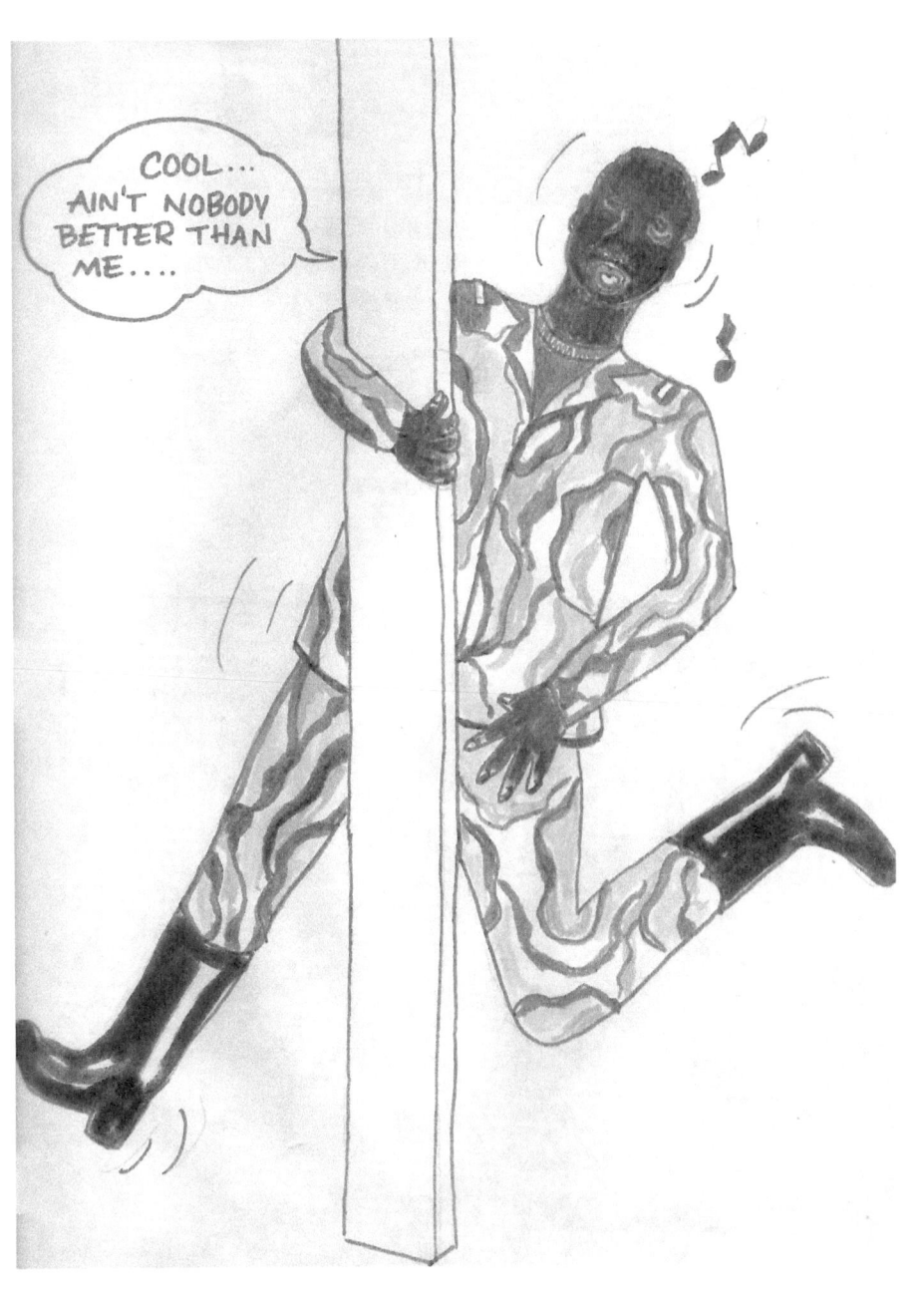

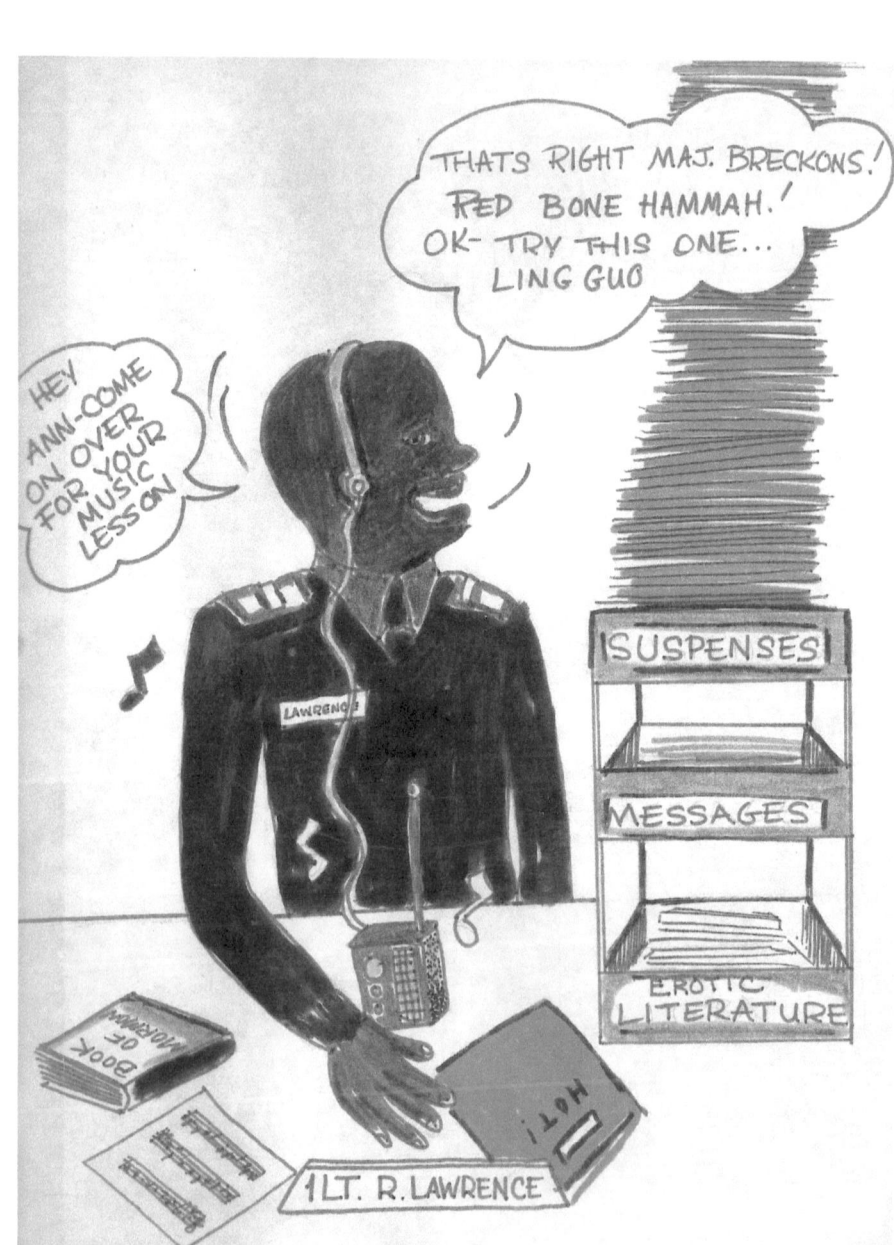

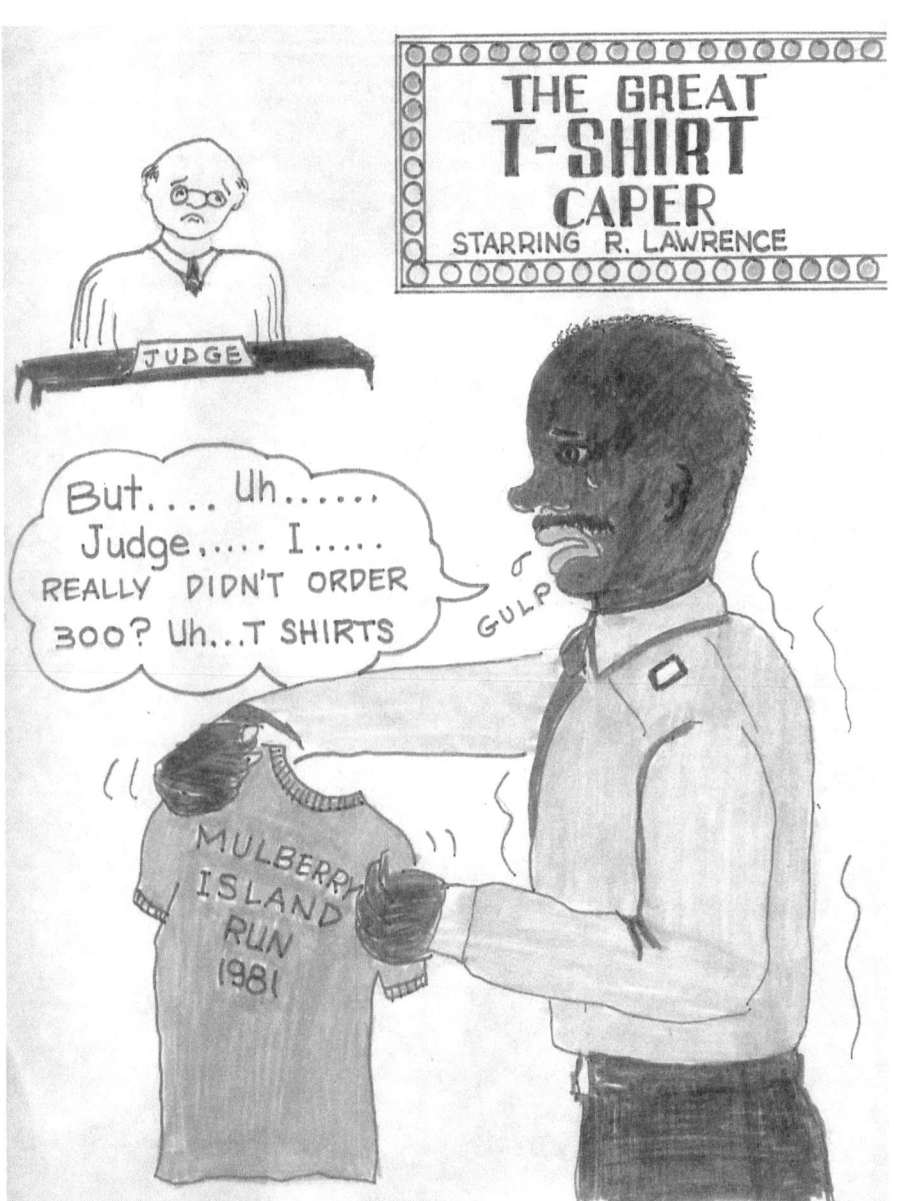

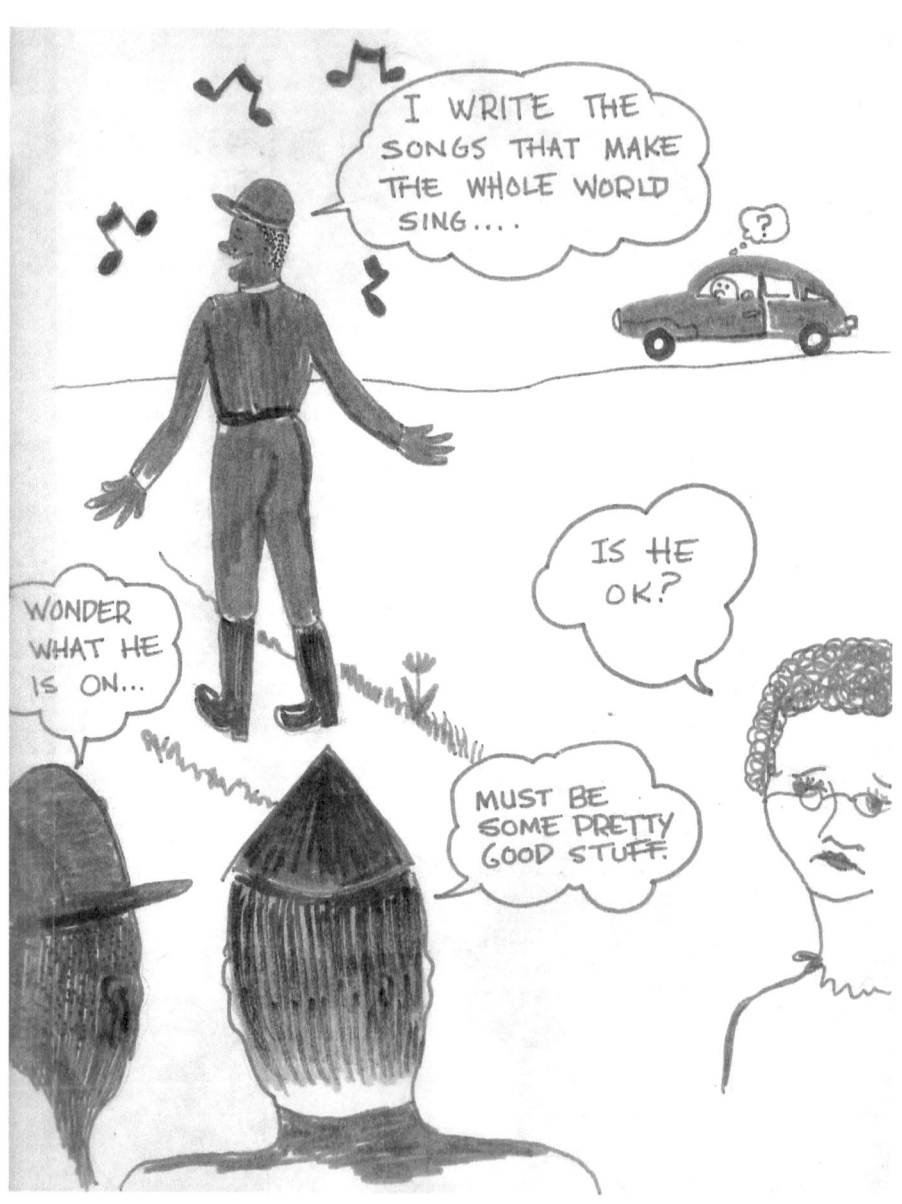

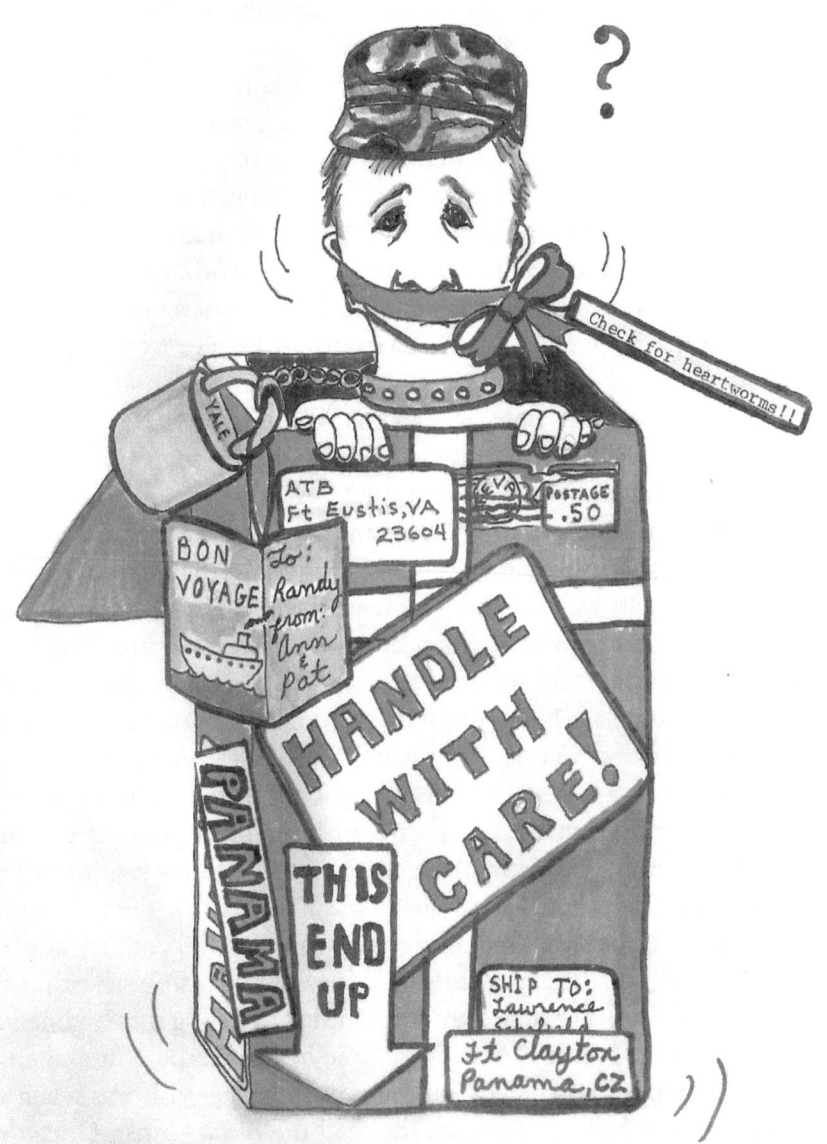

After a spectacular send-off from Fort Eustis, we descended upon the 193rd Infantry Brigade in Panama. There, I served as the executive officer of the Headquarters Company and the first platoon leader in the Mad Dog Alpha Company in the 4/10 Battalion located on the Atlantic side of Panama at Fort Davis. After being "too mean to live and too tough to die," I branch transferred to the Finance Corps. In Panama, we lived on Fort Davis in an old Generals' Quarters converted into a duplex. We had the upstairs, and the rooms were huge. There were three large bedrooms and two bathrooms, with a combination living/dining room with a dimension of eighteen by thirty-six feet. Panama was a great tour because Celinda and I got into verbal altercations periodically throughout the three years and resolved issues without family input. Plus we had live-in maids so there were no disagreements in reference to housework. In addition, this is where we both started acting and producing entertainment for the military community. Celinda was a character in *Sylvia Plat* and *The Owl and the Pussycat* and was Slim in *Snow White Goes West* and El Galo in *The Fantastic*. Stars were born in Panama. Celinda was also the Sunday school superintendent. While out running with the chaplain, I was hit by the mirror of a van traveling 45 miles per hour passing another car, which required several stitches to put me back together again. Lamarr and Jason were growing rapidly and developing into their own individual personalities. Lamarr was not really motivated when it came to homework, and Jason made this comment when he was in preschool after witnessing the riding Lamarr was receiving after school, "Dad, Mom, you don't have to do me like Lamarr. I am going to do my schoolwork," and he did forever!

Also, during our adventure in Panama, Mattie and her new beau Ralph came to visit. It was a jam-packed week, and I got the opportunity to show a country and culture that I had grown to love. Three months before it was time for us to have a permanent change of station back to the states, Daddy and Jessa Bell came for a visit. It was Daddy's first time out of the United States, and he displayed all signs of enjoying the country and the people. Jessa Bell was her usual mean and jealous self, from shutting the door on Daddy's leg every time they enter the car to hating the Panamanian sales lady who flirted with Daddy every time he visited the post exchange. The only moment of peace between them during their visit was when we took them to Portobello to a church that had the Black Christ. Once they walked into the church, they both just stared at the Christ figure and sat down in the pews next each other with look of peace and serenity.

In June 1985, we came back to the United States, to Fort Benjamin Harrison, Indiana, to attend the Finance Officer Advance Course. It was good to be back in the home of the brave, but with it came much misfortune. Mama Sue, my maternal grandmother, died and what a gut-wrenching experience. The moment I got the call, I cried until I left the airport in Norfolk with Olivia and Ronald. Mama Sue's death took so much out of me. She was the real mother that I did not have growing up. She always made me feel like someone special and was there for me through all of my growing pains. What an irreplaceable void. We were there only six months, and it was great because Celinda and the boys got to experience the magic of Indianapolis, Indiana. We had a nice little townhouse that actually had the washer and dryer upstairs. We really got into the Indianapolis culture and found ourselves eating out every Friday night, which was quite an ordeal trying to find a restaurant that did not have a long line waiting to get a table.

In January 1986, at thirty-two years old, I attended Airborne School back at Fort Benning, Georgia, which nearly killed me. I managed to make it through ground and tower week without my heart bursting. On my first jump from the airplane, I broke my ankle, so they made me complete one more jump that day to confirm the break. Aided by cast, crutches, and my 1973 Nova, we arrived into Fort Stewart, Georgia, to join Celinda and our sons. While stationed at Fort Stewart, Mom Mattie died in early 1987. I experienced another significant loss, an instrumental part of my growing into manhood. In addition, during my tenure at Fort Stewart, while we were visiting home, I encountered one of the most frightening experiences. Celinda, the kids, and I were staying on the Colony Timeshare Resort on Thirteenth Street and Atlantic Avenue. Late one evening, I was returning to the condo and entering through the gate off Boardwalk. Just as I was using my key to open the gate, I felt something on the back of my head and heard the words, "Don't move or say a thing or I will blow your goddamn head off! Now give me your wallet." I froze in my tracks, and he took my wallet out of my right rear pocket and took off running. It took me few seconds to regain my composure, and as I started my search for this criminal, I ran into a policeman on duty. After a brief explanation of what just occurred, he told me to get into the police van, and I rode around with him for a few minutes up and down the strip to see if we could find my assailant. Unfortunately, we had no luck, so the police officer took my report. I went upstairs to the condo and told Celinda about my near-death experience, and she suggested that I call my sister Olivia. While talking to Olivia, I had a surge of emotion and erupted into tears. She really helped me to put things into prospective and deal with the issue at hand. They did not catch this guy, even though he used my phoned card to make numerous long distance calls.

At Fort Stewart, initially I held the position as the chief of pay and examination, which included the travel, accounting, disbursing, and the in/ out processing sections, supervising more than 200 civilians and soldiers. I loved that job, until we received a new finance and accounting officer. He began making changes in the personnel at the different supervisory levels, which strongly appeared to be racially motivated. Unfortunately, I was not able to hold my tongue, and finally I did something that was elevated to the general's attention, and he immediately fired me. I was told to clean out of my office and go home for signing a check for a service member that was leaving within the hour for a permanent change of station, which was validated through a check writing machine that was not functioning properly during the distribution period. I sat home for two weeks before the personnel department was able to make a placement. I was hurt and sent letters to *Oprah* and *60 Minutes* in hopes that they would expose this injustice. Well, *60 Minutes* flat out refused and *Oprah* let me down easy. I kept both letters and have included them below. I think Oprah really did sign the letter herself.

CBS/BROADCAST GROUP

CBS Inc., 51 West 52 Street
New York, New York 10019
(212) 975-3166

Marjorie Holyoak, Director
Audience Services

·Dear Mr. Lawrence: June 3, 1988

I am replying to your request that 60 MINUTES investigate a matter
about which you are concerned.

We regret to learn of the difficulties you are facing, but must inform
you that, after careful consideration, 60 MINUTES has decided not to
report on them. As you know, each edition of 60 MINUTES is limited
to only three subjects, which must be selected from among dozens that
could conceivably -- and justifiably -- be explored. The staff cannot
investigate any matters not selected for on-air reports, as they must
concentrate their efforts and resources on preparing broadcast material.

Although we cannot help you, we hope that you will find assistance
through other avenues.

Cordially,

M. Holyoak

Mr. Randy Lawrence
Route 3, Box 101E Wells Road
Hinesville, GA 31313

CBS/Broadcast Group: CBS Television Network,
CBS Entertainment, CBS Sports, CBS News, CBS Television Stations,
CBS Radio, CBS Operations and Engineering

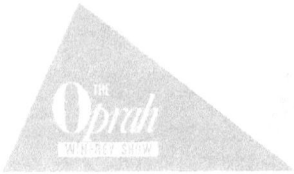

P.O. BOX 909715 CHICAGO, ILLINOIS 60690

May 17, 1988

Dear Randy,

Thank you so much for suggesting a topic
for *The Oprah Winfrey Show*. We welcome
new ideas or new angles to old ideas.

I've forwarded your letter to our producers
for their review. Thanks for sharing your
thoughts and for watching.

Best wishes,

Oprah Winfrey

P.S. Thanks for sharing your story.

They sent me over to run the Army Emergency Relief Office. I hit the ground running and was able to combine my money management skills and deep compassion to aid soldiers and their families in financial distress. I really excelled at making the Army Emergency Relief Office run smooth and efficiently. So good that my immediate supervisor let me write my own Officer Evaluation Report. Boy did I need that to restore my somewhat damaged ego!

Celinda came up with a bright idea of expanding the family, so we adopted a little five-year-old girl, Stephanie Amy Lawrence, in December 1987. I requested another overseas tour, so in September 1988, we moved to Berlin, Germany. What a time to experience Germany before, during, and after the fall of the Berlin Wall. Celinda and I both managed to obtain master's degrees during my tenure in Berlin. I attended Boston University and received a Master of Education with a concentration in Counseling. Berlin was the best tour of duty of all of my military assignments. There was so much personal growth and eye-opening experiences. In December 1991, I was transferred back to Fort Monroe, Virginia, and bought a house in Virginia Beach. On July 31, 1992, I accepted an early retirement package, the Voluntary Separation Agreement. I made my mad exit from Uncle Sam, taking the money and running right into employment with the Virginia Beach City Public Schools as a guidance counselor at a brand-new school named Tallwood High School. During the summer of 1994, Stephanie went to live with her foster mother in Swainsboro, Georgia. That's my brief history, and now it's time for the reason I decided to tell my story.

Chapter 2

Discovery

I was stretched out naked across our brass king size bed while hot chocolate fingers were touching and probing my anatomy. Every touch ignited the walls of my circulatory system, which manifested into a blood rush straight to the private dancer. I was receiving a physical examination from an intelligent, sexy, creative, and warm-spirited lady who possessed a grand sense of humor; she had the most beautiful captivating large brown eyes. This lovely lady was none other than Celinda; my wife of seventeen years. Celinda was attending Norfolk State University (NSU) School of Nursing to become a registered nurse. I must add that she was already a registered respiratory therapist and possessed a degree in bachelor of science in biology and a master's degree in hospital administration. As she explored the different areas of my anatomy, stirring up my desire, she simultaneously provided a detailed explanation of her actions, which intensified the blood rush. The eroticism rapidly dissipated when Celinda discovered a small lump under my right arm. The sparkle in her loving brown eyes immediate changed to a look of concern and fear of the unknown. After explaining the lymphatic system and functions, she suspected that the lump was an inflamed lymphoid. She said that the small growth the size of a pea tucked away in my armpit was not normal. She strongly recommended that I speak with my primary care physician. I had an appointment already scheduled to see Dr. Voss at the end of June and felt that would be a good time to address my concerns. I was not pressed with this discovery, for I was already in a humbled state from dealing with diabetes since September 1990. I was confident even then that whatever the diagnosis of this growth would reveal, I would deal with it too!

On the morning of June 22, 1995, I got into my calm mode to face the Hampton Roads tunnel traffic. Maneuvering in that traffic could make one crazy if you allowed yourself to become a part of the rush hour madness and attitudes of the road-raged drivers. Upon arriving at the Veteran's Hospital, I felt pretty good about seeing Dr. Voss. I was finally making progress in bringing my glucose control to an acceptable level. I managed to control my diabetes through diet and exercise the first three years after being diagnosed. Things went a little haywire upon returning home from Europe with three kids and no spouse. We lived in Berlin for a little over three years, and my relationship with Celinda was on and off during that period, so she opted to stay in Berlin. I came home with the kids on Friday, December 13, 1991, to start a new spouseless life. Upon returning to the United States, three life-changing events came on the scene—career change, filing for a divorce, and planning for my wedding with another woman. Anyway, that's another book; however, it was the inception of my diabetes spiraling out of control. It was a roller coaster trip finding the correct insulin dosage, through trial and error, that would work best with my body type and lifestyle. Dr. Voss's small shapely figure, wavy blonde hair, and Bette Davis blue eyes made it easy for me to stay focused and follow her advice. In addition, Dr. Voss possessed exceptional medical knowledge. Her deep compassion, coupled with her great bedside manner, and knowing her patients were qualities that always made my visits to the Veteran's Hospital a pleasant experience. After reviewing my blood work and a gentle tongue lashing about my overall state of glucose control, Dr. Voss instructed me to hop up on her examination table so she could check out the lump under my right arm. Her first response was "Hmm this sure is big," which she repeated several times. Then she stated, "I am not sure what this is; however, lets monitor this closely and see if gets any bigger." Since there was no pain attached to the pea-sized lump, I left in good spirits and didn't give it another thought for at least a couple of months.

Summer arrived, and I did my usual bum time. Daily, I would awake before 6:00 a.m., don my biking apparel, and ride ten miles to the oceanfront. This time also awarded me the opportunity to fire up old vocal cords. I would belt out quite a few songs during the joyous riding time. From time to time, on my bike rides, I would bring the lyrics to a song to commit the words to memory and iron out the kinks in the melody while pedaling my ass off. The combination of the physical activity and singing my heart out always filled my spirits with jubilation. Once reaching the boardwalk, I would ride to its end, dismount my bicycle, and walk with my bike rolling by my side while experiencing the peace that the beach atmosphere always provided. At Twenty-second Street, I would lock my bike, strip down to my biking shorts, and take a plunge into the Atlantic Ocean. The salted water coupled with the motion of the waves slapping my body around had a unique way of dismantling my woes. Once the cleansing dip was over, I would return to the boardwalk and sit on one of the benches. There, I would listen to the sound of the beach coming alive with people; periodically, a homeless person or a wino would join me on the bench, and we would share life experiences through dialogue. Something about their lifestyle has always been truly intriguing, even though they appeared to have a grand sense of freedom or in a wino's case all of their cares of the world temporarily eased. My high moments of sharing with them did not manifest into the idea of trading places. The bike ride home would be equally as fulfilling as I sang every mile of the way.

I would return to the house at around 10:30 a.m., and then I would head out to Bally Total Fitness Center and on alternating days spend at least an hour and a half on my lightweight training/sauna and an hour on the days that consisted swimming six laps, sitting in whirlpool, and sauna. Believe it or not, if there were no other people around, I would sing for the acoustics of the shower, sauna, and pool/whirlpool areas were out this world. The sound was definitely music to my ears; however, the moment a human form presented itself, I immediately killed the notes even in the middle of a climax. Once home from the gym, most of time I did something with the kids. Being a good father to Lamarr (Mars), sixteen years old, and Jason (Vater), fourteen years old, was at the top of my list of things fueling my existence. Stephanie (Miss Butt), twelve years old, was living in Swainsboro, Georgia, with the Habershams since the summer of 1993 (again another book). Having the summer off really gave me time to get the desire to be a bum out of system and to recharge my soul so that returning to work always had a high level of excitement.

The Saturday before Labor Day was our annual Lawrence Day at Munden Point Park. My siblings and I would plan a very eventful day and split the cost eight ways. There would usually be more than one hundred relatives and friends in attendance. There was enough food to feed an army, with barbecued pig and fried chicken from Breeze Inn as the center food attraction. Oh, and please don't let me forget the most important food item that sometimes would cause an altercation if someone was deprived of this morsel of delight—Celinda's famous sour cream pound cake and utterly delicious fourteen carrot cake. Literally, some people would become unglued if they were not awarded the opportunity to partake one of those taste bud dancers. There was something for everyone—play ground, basketball, volleyball, horse shoes, baseball, and bingo with prizes for the old folks, or you can just walk out and enjoy the atmosphere of the James River. This day always made Daddy feel good because his children could provide such a wonderful day to people with a charge, and there was plenty of leftover food for them to take home.

This was definitely a special day for me too. I had the opportunity to interact with so many people that had a tremendous impact on my development. I could always count on hearing my favorite line from my Grandmother Mattie's two first cousins Cut'in Bessie and Cut'in May. I was just being myself using my sense of humor on the older ladies and before I knew it, the line rolled off like music to my ears. Cut'in May said "Lord Bessie, I declare Randy's crazy!" And Bessie responded in her high soprano voice "Na he ain't May, he's a fool!" God I loved those ladies; they were so good to me during my adolescence. Their wisdom and candor permeate my existence. The day was filled with physical activity, good food, and immense laughter. It was also a time when my extended family could see what a beautiful person Celinda was and the magical chemistry between us. Lamarr and Jason got a chance to get know more of their relatives and have even more fun with their first cousins.

School started after Labor Day, and I was in my usual state of ecstasy after a wonderful and restful summer. This was the beginning of my fourth year as a guidance counselor at Tallwood High School and the end of my employment probationary period. Mr. Morgan, our school's principal, would always ask me from time to time, "Randy, when are you going to start working around here?" I would always respond with the day I start working around here will be the day that I quit. We shared a hardy laugh after that brief interaction. Now that I was free at last, I told Mr. Morgan that he had not seen anything yet and that I was going to bust loose this year since I was no longer on probation.

Upon receiving my first Leave and Earnings Statement from the beginning of my fourth year of employment, I noticed that one day of sick leave was subtracted by mistake. I immediately brought it to the attention of Mary our attendance clerk and commented in a joking fashion that I may need that day for a real illness. Little did I know that what we speak with our lips will come to pass in time. I went on about the usual business at school. I had died and gone to heaven being employed at Tallwood High School. Tallwood was a new school that opened in August 1992, and I was fortunate enough to be picked by Mr. Morgan to join the original faculty and staff. Mr. Morgan with his administrators did a fantastic job of selecting faculty members to staff Tallwood High School, the home of the Mighty Lions. Mr. Morgan's number one criterion for being selected was that one would have to embrace his philosophy of loving and being there for the kids. Mr. Morgan, a charismatic leader (who loved to kiss and hug), created a school environment for our students that promoted academic and athletic excellence while simultaneously embracing diversity and all ethnicities. I was filled with excitement every morning and was always looking forward to a new adventure. Every day at Tallwood was unique, and laughter was no stranger to the majority of my workday.

Then one night, the last of September, with my arms up and behind my head waiting for Celinda to join me in bed, I noticed her beautiful large brown eyes swelled with tears focused on my right armpit. She asked if I were experiencing any pain and if I had noticed the size of the lump now protruding from my armpit. I responded with no and then had a look myself and was amazed for the lump was the size of oval-shaped fifty-cent coin. She then demanded that I make an appointment with my primary care physician through my health maintenance organization Optima insurance immediately. I took heed to her request and made an appointment with Dr. Petal the next day, which was the last Monday in September. Upon arriving to Dr. Petal's office, I knew that I was in for at least a forty-five-minute wait after I was subjected to the cold and uncaring demeanor of his receptionist due to my existence in their facility. However, once I got to see Dr. Petal, my human existence rapidly reappeared. Dr. Petal always had a way of making me feel like I was his most important patient. Once we got through the usual physical examination procedures, he stated, "I don't know what that lump is, so I am going to refer you to a surgeon." He wrote a referral, made an appointment with Dr. Rahman for Wednesday of the same week, and sent me on my way.

On Wednesday morning, I entered Dr. Rahman's reception area. There were about seven other people waiting for the doctor. I received a warm greeting from the receptionist and was asked to complete some demographic and medical history information on myself. I sat nervously, and while completing the forms, I listened to the conversation of the people in the waiting room. The comments were all favorable, and everyone seemed to sing praises for Dr. Rahman for he was known as a surgeon with incredible precision. I thought that I would be there for hours on end; however, it was only about forty-five minutes before my name was called. Dr. Rahman, a man of Indian descent, asked me to undress so that he could examine the area of concern. Once on his examination table, he felt the lump under my arms, examined my abdomen area, and then asked when was the last time I had a rectal exam. When I responded in July 1992, my exit medical physical examination from the army, he requested that I lay on my side; he slid on a latex glove and with his hand penetrated my anus with what felt like the biggest finger in the world. My army exit physical examination, which included a rectal examination, was not nearly as invasive, I guess because I had a female physician with small fingers. However, this time, it was quite uncomfortable and borderline pain. These stimulated a suppressed memory of my first sexual experience at twelve years old, which left a horrible mental scar. Once the rectal examination was complete, Dr. Rahman requested that I get dressed and return to his consultation office. I sat next to him at his desk, and he said, "See my assistant out front and she will schedule a surgery appointment this Friday." Puzzled, I asked what my options were. He responded, "I don't know what the lump is, and you don't either, so let's take it out and find out what it is." Now that's what I call straight to the point. So I followed his instructions.

I went back to work and came home as usual. During that time, Mars, my eldest son, was a senior and Vader was a sophomore at Tallwood High School. Since we lived in Green Run, the boys were attending Tallwood High School out of zone. In the mornings, Lamarr and Jason would ride to school together in our blue 1992 Pontiac Grand Am four-door sedan. That afternoon, Lamarr was dismissed early from school because he had a part-time employment with the Office of Leadership School Activities section, and Jason rode home with me in the royal blue 1954 210 series Chevrolet two-door sedan. That 54 was my baby; it was the first and only car I purchased on a Visa credit card. I remember it like it was yesterday. I had been eyeing this striking vehicle on the front lot of the Acura Dealer on Holland Road for two months. Then one day in May 1992, I drove by and the 54 was parked at the back of the lot. I made a mad U-turn and rapidly entered the Acura Dealer's parking lot. I went over to the 54 and at first glance up close, the love and desire bubbled inside as I checked out her sweet curves and the condition of her interior. A sales representative named Mike approached me and asked if I was interested in purchasing this classic automobile. I responded with depends on how much? Then he said, "Make me an offer?" I said jokingly $2,500. He said, "It's yours!" I said, "do you take Visa or Master Card?" He replied "Yes!" I drove my new/old royal blue 1954 Chevrolet 210 series two-door sedan home that evening. The rest is the start of a thrilling challenge to the world of restoration and a whole new story.

Anyway, let's get back to home life. Our daily weekday routine consisted of after Jason and I arriving home from school, I would prepare dinner. Celinda was working as a respiratory therapist at Maryview Hospital in Portsmouth while attending NSU in the evening, so it was a while before she would get home in the evenings. By the time dinner was prepared, Mars would be home from his part-time employment. That evening at dinner, I shared the news with the boys about the day I met with Dr. Rahman, and business went on as usual. Dinner is something we always shared together, and it was a peaceful time to share stuff along with telling jokes. We always had classical or opera (mostly Giacomo Puccini) music playing in the background to keep things calm at the table. We discovered earlier with the kids that R&B would make us jam at the table. When Celinda arrived later that evening, I had dinner waiting for her and sat at the kitchen table and discussed my new adventure. She said that she would take off from work to accompany me on Friday for the surgery. This would be my first experience with any type of surgery so ambivalence ran rapidly through my psyche.

Friday morning, I rolled out bed feeling great as usual; however, things were just a little crazy because this morning I would ride to school with Lamarr and Jason. They normally left home much later than I did. I would be at school no later 6:30 a.m. every morning and my sons did not usually leave home until 7:00 a.m., so that meant I would have to walk in with the students arriving, and on those rare occasions when I did do that, it would make me crazy and be extremely difficult to get on track for a fast-paced multitask job. This day, I adjusted relatively well, and before I could get into the flow of things, Celinda was there to take me to Chesapeake General Hospital. We arrived at the hospital, received a painless check in, and in the blink of an eye I was on a gurney being prepped for surgery. I looked in the eyes of the anesthesiologist and ask if he was going to explain to me what I was about to experience. He replied with a smile, "Mr. Lawrence I'm going to explain everything to you" as he lowered a cup over my nose and mouth. That was the last thing I heard until the sound of my cough, making me realize that I was waking up from the deep sleep. The waking up process from being put to sleep was terrifying. Fear entered my soul as I vehemently battled to return to a conscious state. I felt like I could not get out of the sleep mode. There was no pain involved, just a feeling of being locked in a horrible dream. Finally, after what seemed like ten minutes, the natural feelings entered my body. After the natural feeling resumed totally, I noticed Celinda sitting there by my bedside with sad eyes and a smile on her face asking if I were all right. I told her now I am and explained what I just experienced.

The day was still young, so I was discharged from the hospital, with a word to phone Dr. Rahman's office for an immediate follow-up visit. What a grand sight 3712 Seven Springs Court home sweet home was to return to. Once inside, I slowly climbed the stairs headed for the bed for more rest and to make a quick phone call to schedule a follow-up appointment. While speaking with Dr. Rahman's assistant, she said (I am sure it slipped out), "Hmm he doesn't normally see patients back so soon after surgery; oh! I mean can you come in on Monday morning at 10:00 a.m.?" I agreed that would be a good time, hung up the phone, and slowly fell into a restful sleep.

Saturday was a normal day for the kids and me. However, that Sunday morning, my sons and I had preregistered for the American Diabetes six-mile walkathon. So off to Hampton we went for I wasn't feeling any pain from the surgery and need to get out and get a breath of fresh air. The walk went well, both Mars and Vader finished before I did. We received medals and nice completion certificates. Doing things like that with my sons always gave me a warm fuzzy feeling inside. We returned home for Sunday dinner, and all was well in the Lawrence home one more time. Sunday evening, I was trying to understand the extraordinarily good treatment from Celinda and slowly entered dreamland. Monday after completing my daily morning hygiene rituals, which consist of nine S's (shout, stretch, stick, shit, shower, shave, swallow, and shoot all while singing; I know you are wondering what stick, sallow, and shoot means: stick my fingers to get a glucose reading, swallow my vitamins, and shoot to take my insulin injections), and last but not the least apply coco butter lotion to my ashy body. Once rejuvenated, I grabbed a quick breakfast and fired up the 54. I arrived at school at 6:30 a.m. and prepared for a much welcomed invasion of the young people. Celinda came around 9:15 a.m., and we were off in flash to meet my new destiny.

This time the wait was not long. We were there only about fifteen minutes before we entered the door embarking on a new opportunity. Dr. Rahman looked at Celinda and me and stated, "The lymphoid that I removed on Friday was malignant. You have cancer, so I am going to make an appointment for you to see an oncologist for treatment. Additionally, you have double hernia; however, we will deal with that after we treat the cancer." So there it was, I really didn't expect to hear that; however, I was at peace. I knew that dealing with diabetes for the last five years had already made me a very humble man. Celinda's eyes were glassy from the moment we entered Dr. Rahman's office. Once we were in the black 94 Chevrolet Impala SS, Celinda grabbed the steering wheel and started to cry hysterically, which I responded with, "Celinda, maybe I should drive because I would like to live to experience whatever treatments are in store for me. The state that you are in right now, we will be lucky if we make home alive." With that said, she pulled herself together and took me back to school. At school, I shared the good news with my guidance director, Gay Dailey, and eventually the information trickled down to my other colleagues. I definitely felt a sense of sadness in the guidance office that day, but my spirit remained in a joyful joking mood. I guess the biggest obstacle for me at moment was the unknown, for that really played on my mind. What test will I have to have? What will the treatments consist of? Even though I knew I could meet any challenge live or die, the fear factor of the unknown was prevalent in my mind.

Chapter 3

Oncologist Recommendations

Dr. Baskhir Rao was his name, and treating cancer was his claim to fame. My first meeting with him was straightforward with no fluffy words in his presentation. Dr. Rao said that without any treatment, I might have a maximum life expectancy of five years, and with treatment, chances are I could return to my normal life expectancy. He said before he could develop a treatment plan, there were a few more tests that I needed to complete to determine the progression my new friend Hodgkin's diseases. These extra tests prescribed include a chest x-ray, complete body scan (MRI), and bone marrow removal procedure. His administrative assistant, Cindy, scheduled appointments for a series of medical events to add to my life experiences.

The chest x-ray was simple and not strange to an army veteran. However, the MRI was a different story. I was given a thick green liquid to drink, and upon consumption, it provided a flavor that was unique to my tongue thirty minutes prior to launching time. Once my stomach was bloated from the tasty thick green liquid, I was ushered into a room that contains a machine that looked like a giant donut with a tongue extended. The technician asked me to lie on what I described as the long tongue and started explaining what to expect. He said that after injecting an IV in my right arm, he will start feeding iodine into my veins to assist the giant donut in capturing accurate pictures my total body's current landscape. In addition, he stated that once the iodine starts to penetrate my system, I would begin feel warm all over. Then the action commenced. What an understatement on his part. He was definitely right about feeling warm all over; however, my testicles felt like they were on fire. This made me very uncomfortable, and my stomach started to rumble as my body was slowing going through the giant donut. Nausea prevailed, and I began to erupt like a hot explosive volcano. The technician rapidly grabbed some paper towels and started to wipe up what he could and said, "Mr. Lawrence, we are almost finished, so please just lay still and we will get you clean up as soon this test is completed." I laid there a couple of minutes, which seemed more like a couple of days in my sea of volcanic aftermath with two burning balls of fire. In my deliberation during that moment, the five-year life expectancy was sounding like a viable option. Once I was all cleaned up, I went to the waiting room where my eldest sister Olivia was waiting for me and inquired about my MRI experience. She asked, "How did things go?" I replied other than my nuts being on fire and throwing up, things went pretty good!

The bone marrow removal was definitely an experience that I do not care to ever repeat. Olivia accompanied me on this venture too. We arrived at Bayside Hospital, and I was immediately taken up to a different floor to be prepped for the procedure. There I was lying on a table with my buttocks exposed while Dr. Rao and a couple of nurses proceeded to talk me through the process. After the injection, my butt became numb. I felt nothing until Dr. Rao state that he had piece of bone marrow that he would remove and that I may experience some discomfort. When he said "here we go," the extreme intense pain lasted less than a second, totally infiltrating every part of my physical human form which manifested into tears shooting out of my eyes. Dr. Rao began to boast about the size of the bone marrow that came out when he made the extraction. He and his nurses were singing praises while I lay there with my buttocks exposed and deliberating what just happen? Once all the excitement was over from the extraction of the small piece of bone marrow, Dr. Rao ask me to get dressed and check out of the hospital. In addition, Dr. Rao instructed me to call Cindy to schedule an appointment to go over my treatment plan. I got dressed and went to the patient waiting area, and there was the effulgent smile of Olivia waiting for me to hear my experience and take me home.

My family and extended family were overly concerned about what the treatments entailed. So my sisters Olivia, Barbara Sue, Patsy, Mattie, and Frances, Daddy's fourth wife Mama B, and Mattie's girlfriend Yvonne accompanied Celinda and me to the appointment to see Dr. Rao. Cindy had a strange look on her face when the entourage entered the office. They told her that they were there for support and this way they could receive first-hand information regarding my treatments. Dr. Rao came out and said that he was ready to go over the treatment and commanded Cindy to find chairs so that everyone could fit in his office.

Once we were all seated and introductions were completed, Dr. Rao proceeded with his diagnosis and treatment plan. He stated that I was in stage one of Hodgkin's disease, which is 100% curable with proper treatment. He recommended radiation treatments and scheduled an appointment at the Sentara Cancer Center in Norfolk. In addition, he recommended that I visit my dentist before I start any treatments. The entourage was all happy with this news and expressed praises to the Lord and stated that they would be here for me every step of the way. My mind set at that moment was how blessed I was to have been born into such a wonderful family and that I can do this! I must add that my siblings have always been a tremendous source of my strength. All through the years, they have provided unconditional love and support.

Chapter 4

Radiation Up Top Time!

I indeed paid a visit to my dentist, Dr. Schiff. Dr. Schiff did not have the warmest demeanor; however, I appreciated his straightforwardness coupled with pearly white teeth, so he definitely had my trust. He made a mold of my teeth and prescribed a fluoride gel to squeeze into the plastic teeth mold and placed over my teeth during radiation treatments. A few days after my visit with Dr. Schiff, Celinda and I were off to the Sentara Cancer Center in Norfolk to meet with my radiation doctor. After about fifteen minutes of waiting, we were taken to the examination room, and a few minutes later Dr. Walker and another doctor (I have forgotten her name, but man did she have some delicious beautiful large brown eyes) walked in. I felt an instant connection with Dr. Walker, who possessed a grand sense of humor, and immediately I knew that I was in great hands. With a cross communication of exchanges lined with jokes and tremendous humor between Dr. Walker and myself, he managed to convey a treatment plan consisting of receiving a total of forty radiation treatments, twenty on the chest area and twenty on the abdomen and below. He scheduled me for radiation treatments Monday through Friday at 3:00 p.m. I told him that I was still trying to get my diabetes back in control and needed to lose some weight. He said that we should concentrate on getting rid of the cancer and besides I would need that extra weight down the road. That was a first, a doctor telling me it was OK to be overweight. He also stated that if I wanted to father more children, I should make a deposit in the sperm bank plus I had to discontinue using deodorant. He was detailed in his explanation of my treatments and what to expect physically once I started radiation. Celinda expressed to Dr. Walker that she was currently working full time and would like for him to sign a letter for her employer requesting that she work part time so that she could take care of me, which he agreed to do. With that, we were off once again in wild anticipation of my future endeavors.

Meanwhile, at work I tried to keep a low profile. Tallwood was a place that had already experienced many tragedies from deaths to terminal illness. Being a relatively new school, the Tallwood family was no stranger to adversities. I shared the news with Mr. Morgan and asked him not to put it out to the faculty or the students. Mr. Morgan asked, "What can we do?" I responded with just make me laugh as much as possible. In addition, I shared the Big "C" diagnosis with Gay. When I expressed to Gay how very concerned I was about not being able wear deodorant because I profusely sweat and sometimes the greatest smells encompassed in a liquid form were excreted from my skin. She then replied, "Hell Ran, the rest of us will stop wearing deodorant so they won't know who smells in the department." We had a hearty laugh and knew that sooner than later, everyone would learn of the Big "C," and as the news trickled down, the sad eyes permeated my atmosphere.

As a family, we were members of the Virginia Stage Association. Once a month, we would usher at the Wells Theater in Norfolk. Celinda and I always worked together on the left doors of the orchestra section or collected tickets at the main entrance doors. Lamarr and Jason work upstairs on each door to the mezzanine section. This was a good bonding time for the family. Over the years, all of the productions were really good and some were outstanding. We got to see all of the productions, which always resulted in thorough critique on the drive back home. I always felt a high level of excitement facing and exchanging comments with Celinda in reference to patrons. Most of the time, we always agreed with a smile and eye gestures regarding a brief description of the characters that entered the foyer. We had a ministry for all of eccentric behaviors exhibited by the people in attendance. Lamarr and Jason always enjoyed ushering when two old gentlemen would usher with us. They were just two lively men, and the boys called the one with a hunchback Mortermore. They usually worked upstairs with Lamarr and Jason. The first of October, we ushered for "Blite Spirit" by Noel Coward.

Friday, October 13, 1995, was opera night. The opera was another activity that Celinda and I shared a passion for. Let me digress for a moment and take you back to first time we discovered this undying passion. I had always enjoyed opera music but had not had the experience of attending a full opera. We were living in Berlin, and a lady in my office name Manuela Frietag asked me if I were interested in attending an opera. I jumped at the opportunity, and she purchased two tickets for Celinda and me. In addition, she lent us the album of the opera with English translation. Celinda and I listened to the music first, and we knew in that instance it was love. The mellifluous sounds of the orchestra and the opera singers gave me an incredible tingle through my soul. On January 26, 1989, I was downstairs at Biberstieg 6, patiently waiting for the love of my life to come down the stairs. She slowly came down the stairs, eyeing her pumps and long brown legs, slowly appearing with each step until she was totally into my view. I wanted to jump her bones in that instant for her look was truly intoxicating. I managed to regain my composure, and we were off to our first opera. We arrived in the parking garage, and remember just how far my chest was stuck out when I opened the door and that gorgeous lady step out and grabbed my arm. We entered the Deutsche Opera Berlin and were seated in the orchestra second row center stage. When I sat down, there was a German lady beside me. She looked at me, clutched her purse, and actually sat like that throughout the entire opera. I thought to myself that if we could afford orchestra second row seat, what on earth would I want with her purse. Anyway, the conductor came out with the spotlight on him. As the audience applauded, he took a bow and turned around, and the orchestra commenced playing Giacomo Puccini's *La Boheme*. They music was even more beautiful live. Celinda and I sat there holding hands, feeling the power of the string instruments. Once the curtains opened, I was sold. The stage was so real I felt like I was a part of the production. Rodolfo and Marcello belted out some tantalizing notes, causing Celinda and I to gaze at each other periodically, smiling and feeling the passion. What a powerful trade love story. During the beginning of the second act, Mussetta made her grand entrance coming down these giant stairs leaning to the center of the stage where there was an outdoor restaurant and many small shopping stores. As Mussetta made that sensuous walk down the stairs, even though her face was white, I looked at Celinda and said she can't be white walking light that. Celinda just smiled, and we enjoyed every moment of *La Boheme*. In the end, when Mimi was dying, Mussetta took off here gloves and gave them to Schaunard and Collin to sell to get money for a doctor; her hands were black. I immediately turned to Celinda with that I knew it look in my eyes. She gave a validating look, and we were both in tears at end of the climactic ending with Rodolfo's grief-filled notes in his high tenor saying Mimi! What a night. It was definitely the inception of a journey exploring the world of opera.

Once we moved back to Virginia, I became a subscriber to the Virginia Opera Association and always purchased season tickets for the Harrison Opera House in Norfolk. Unlike in Germany, the English translation appeared at the top of the stage during the productions. So on Friday, October 13, I was downstairs patiently waiting for the lovely and sexy Celinda to appear to attend Guiseppe Verdi's Italian libretto *Rigoletto*. She was worth the wait, and opera date was wonderful, which led to a nice nightcap after we returned home.

It was Halloween, and when I entered the cancer center, the office was decorated with lots of holiday delights such as ghost and goblins and a host of unsightly characters sitting in the waiting room. Later I discovered they were cancer patients going through radiation treatments. I met with Dr. Walker to receive an artistic design on my upper torso from the blue print created from my x-ray of the areas to radiate. I lay lifeless but with a smile on a table while Dr. Walker transcribed the blue print on my chest and back with a permanent marker. This was an inception of the things to come, and I was beginning to feel that this cancer thing just may be real and what a long road I had ahead.

Back at home, we had to make some changes to accommodate this new undertaking. Lamarr still worked at his COE job with the Student Activities Office downtown through his Computer Information Systems class and was leaving school at 12:20 p.m., so Jason started riding home with me in the afternoon. Celinda reduced her work hours, which really cut her bringing home more than $3,000 per month to $185 every two weeks. Of course, the monthly car payment of $450 for the Impala SS was deducted before she received that whooping sum of $185. I thought to myself, how on earth are we going to make it financially when our monthly expenses were right around $6,000? And believe me, my counselor salary and army retirement pay still had us coming up at least $2,000 short every month. What the hell, my health was high priority, and since Celinda was going to take care of me, we would have to find a way to meet our financial obligations. It was decided that Jason would accompany me to my radiation treatments after we got out of school and drive us home afterward. So we were off with this new plan.

The first of November, we did our usher thing at the Wells Theater for the production of *Once on This Island* by Ahers/Flaherty. This proved to be another successful outing under our belts of many. In addition, the first of the month, I went in for my first radiation treatment. After we arrived at the cancer center, I was escorted to a different room while Jason waited patiently in the waiting room. That's when I met Bill, my radiologist. He was a very pleasant young man, and we started with jokes, which always helped me to laugh even during unpleasant situations. He told me to insert the mouth guards, take off my shirt, and get up on the radiation table. Once I was there, he emphasized the importance of being perfectly still. He put in the blue print in the top of the radiation machine and aligned it with the markings on my chest. He flipped the switch, and I heard this microwave sound for about thirty seconds, and then he told me to roll over, and we repeated the same procedure. I thought to myself, gee that was painless, I can do this! It seemed like after every radiation treatment, once I got into the 54, I was overcome with sleep. My head would fall against the door window of the 54 and would be out until we arrived home. Jason was a very safe driver, so I did not have to worry about watching the road.

My weekdays consisted of waking up completing my nine S's, eating breakfast, then firing up the old 54 and off to school, arriving no later than 6:30 a.m. My days at school were always filled with excitement and lots of laughter. It is true that "kids say the darnedest things." I could always count on one of my students saying or doing something to make me laugh. There was never a dull moment at Tallwood, which was good because I did not have time to think about my condition. The students were dismissed each day at 2:00 p.m., so Jason always did his homework until 2:25 p.m., when we promptly head off to the cancer center. Always arriving on time and most of time, there would only be a couple of people waiting with me for the microwave. There were two kids that touched my heart who were in the same predicament. One was a fifteen-year-old Hispanic young man, and English was definitely a second language for him. He managed to smile periodically, but most of the time he displayed painful eyes. I just could not imagine being a teenager and walking his road. Then there this was a five-year-old boy with big blue eyes, no eye brows, and a ball head. Boy was he filled with life. He always came in so happy, with his chest stuck out wearing an effulgent smile, and he always seemed eager to embark on the radiation treatments. His joy was infectious and all encompassing. He was a true inspiration to me. I vowed that if he could be that positive about his incredible challenge at such a young age, then I would join him in exhibiting that wonderful enthusiasm.

Once Jason and I would arrive home, I would prepare dinner. Once Lamarr would arrive home from his job after school, the three of us would have dinner together. Celinda was rarely at home from working part time at the Maryview Hospital, in class at NSU, or studying some place outside of home. After dinner, I would head out to Bally's for a workout. Bally's was always my place to listen to music and sing while I alternated days with a cardiovascular and weight training workouts. I would complete sixty minutes on the stair climber and a 30-minute workout with weights on opposite days. When I would go into the locker room for a shower, I would occasionally get some of the craziest stares because of beautiful markings on my chest and back. One time, a guy asked me if I was in a cult, of course he was a young man. Once I explained my challenge, his face turned red. For some reason, most of the older guys knew that they were markings for cancer treatments and usually inquired about my physical/mental being. Celinda even asked how I could go to gym marked up like that for she would be totally embarrassed. I really didn't even give it a second thought. Physical fitness was a part of my life, and a few markings were not going to stop me from my daily routine.

November 18 was another opera night for us. This time, it was John Strauss II's *Die Fledermaus*. It was in German, so music was hard and cold; however, Celinda and I still managed to get a small buzz. I'm sure that I was getting around at a slower pace before; however, this was when I first realized that the radiation was beginning to affect the way I felt internally and emotionally as well as physically. Even though I was feeling differently, a nightcap was still the order to end the evening.

We started a family tradition once my family returned from overseas. Thanksgiving was at our house. That was the time when our families came together all under one roof. Daddy and Mama B, several of my aunts and uncles, all of my siblings, their children and grandchildren, plus Celinda's parents and some of her siblings and their children would usually attend this time of feasting, fun, and fellowship. Celinda and I spent Thanksgiving Eve preparing the meals. We started this tradition during my early military days. I would prepare the turkey and the main foods that accompanied the meal, while Celinda would bake all of the desserts. Just think when we got married, Celinda was seriously lacking skills in baking and cooking. Celinda picked up my *Betty Crocker Cookbook*, and once we tied the knot, she became an excellent cook. My family members were completely nuts over her pastry and submitted requests whenever they were near our home. That Thanksgiving Eve, just like all the ones before, painted a picture of the two of us burning up the kitchen not just with morsels of delight but with interesting conversations and passionate gestures, relishing our powerful chemistry. Little did I know that I would not experience that level of love and happiness again.

Thanksgiving Day arrived, and our home was filled with family and friends. Some of our extended family members also would bring a dish, making the food plentiful, and so there was always more than enough food that fed sometimes as many as fifty people. And of course Celinda baked her famous sour cream cake and the fourteen carrot cake. We would assemble in the living and dining rooms, join hands ensuring that the circle was intact, and Daddy would offer the blessings. The food was set up in a buffet fashion in the kitchen, and we packed our plates and ate in different rooms in the house until our appetites were more than satisfied. After dinner, we had a talent show as usual. I would always be in charge of this for I would be the emcee, and it would be fantastic to see the different types of talent showcased. My eldest brother, Henry, would always hog the microphone. He loved to sing and did not mine showboating his talent. We followed up with a couple of line dances, the Electric Slide and the Bus Stop. Then, we would break into the gospel mode singing at the top of our lungs "Jesus Can Work It Out" and the "Potter's House" (by my favorite gospel female vocalist Tramaine Hawkins). The young men would go outside to play basketball. The small kids would run through the house, upstairs, outside, or around the house after the talent presentation. For me, I was just happy to have my family and friends share such a special day. Even though I was moving slow during the celebration and singing was not so natural anymore or uncomfortable, I received a blessing and renewed strength and inner peace to what was yet to come.

As I drew closer to the twenty radiation treatments, my spirits elevated. Dr. Walker would have my blood drawn once a week to access the white blood cell count. I had about six treatments left up top when Dr. Walker said that he needed to add four more treatments up top. I was not the happiest camper, but I worked hard on not letting this news dampen my spirits. After every radiation treatment, I started to move slower and slower, so after about three weeks of my body receiving the radiation treatments, I began to move at a snail's pace. In my mind, I was moving fast, but my badly burned internal body was preventing me from reaching my destinations in a timely fashion in which I was accustomed. In fact, people started to notice, especially the students and the faculty at school. Mr. Morgan would come by the office every morning and stick his right foot in the door and shake it around while singing "I feel like busting loose, busting loose." He always knew how make me laugh. I remember running into Ms. Peterson, one of the English teachers in the Guidance Department. She stopped in the hall and said to me, "Boy you have really toned down. I do not hear you singing in hallways anymore." I replied with my cancer challenge and stated that once I completed the treatments, I would get back to my old self. Then she said, "Oh, I was not complaining. I like the new you!" And of course the laughter filled the guidance office. Then there was a time when one of my senior students came by to see me to get a transcript. I jumped out of the chair to complete his request and when I did, I lost my breath and uttered, man I'll be so glad when I get back to normal, and my student said, "Mr. Lawrence, you have never been normal!" I laughed until tears came out of my eyes.

The Tallwood family was caring and supportive as my body started to react to the radiation treatments. There was always a look of concern and a willing outstretched hand. Mrs. Criss, our Fine Department Chair/Art Teacher, painted a beautiful red bird and the Technology Department made a frame. The red bird was surrounded by numerous faculty members with words of encouragement in the boarders of frame. I remember when my colleagues made the presentation of this precious gift to me in my office; I was so overcome with emotion that I was unable to hold back the tears of joy. I hung this picture on what the students called the wall of fame in my office. The wall of fame consisted of old pictures now housing a collage of the students' photos. The special painting now hangs in my bedroom at home.

Well, home life was a little different from school. My extended family was there at every whim or woe from me. My relationship with my siblings and father is a book in itself. The love and support from them was truly overwhelming. My breakdown in support seemed to be stemming from my very own home. I was still preparing all of the meals for the family, plus most evening still had dinner waiting for Celinda. Lamarr and Jason did their own laundry, and I did the rest. In addition, I continued grocery shopping with Lamarr and Jason usually at my side. I was still providing creative financing to make the monthly bill payments and managed to arrive to work on time without taking the time off or missing a day. My relationship with Celinda was turning for the worst and slowly becoming cancer clear. When I say cancer clear, I mean while the cancer was attacking my physical structure and the radiation treatments disarming the cancer, simultaneously my eyes were opening to reexamine my intimate relationship with Celinda.

Then we lost our faithful dog Poochie who had been with us for ten years. Poochie was a mixed breed we called a Heinz 57. We loved Poochie. She was given to us a puppy when we lived in Hinesville, Georgia, and she possessed the sweetest temperament. During the three years we spent living in Europe, Poochie lived with Olivia and Ronald. Ronald Jr. (Boo), my nephew, took very good care of Poochie those three long years. So when we returned to the United States, we were reunited with Poochie and she still remembered all of us well.

In December, my under arm, chest, and back hair fell out. In addition, there was an area in the back of my head that was receiving radiation, and hair fell out too, which looked like two church windows. That radiation was some powerful stuff for I went from my smooth and silky nappy hair to the church window design in the back and wavy in most of the other areas of my head. In fact, when one of my students who was an alumni visited, he asked, "Mr. Lawrence, what do you have going on with your head now? I see naps in the front, waves in the back/sides with fade, and bald in the back." After a gut-retching laugh, I told him about the cancer time. Back in the day, I was known for my creative hairstyles; the newness of being retired from the army hadn't worn off even by then. Mr. Morgan would comment periodically during years, "Randy, you don't know what you want to do with that head of yours, do you?"

Then things began to get really uncomfortable when my neck cracked open due to radiation. My neck look like a burned wound where skin was absent and moist red meat exposed on both sides. When I went to see Dr.

Walker, he made a joke and said, "Hmm, maybe we have given you too much radiation in that area." He recommended that I do not cover this wound, treat it as a burn, and apply an ointment twice a day, which he wrote a prescription to fill. I thought of it as just another beauty mark that adds to my appeal. So I cut the collars out a few shirts to wear to work and started his prescribed regimen.

The stares at school were uncanny, and soon the whole Tallwood family knew the deal. I remember once when I was making a presentation to about one hundred students in the Schola (miniauditorium). When I walked down to the podium, I heard a few gasps from the students, and then there was silence as they looked in amazement at my signature neck. I simply stated with a big smile, I have Hodgkin's disease, a cancer that attacks the lymphatic system, and I am currently receiving radiation treatments; however, since my neck has cracked open, my doctor is going to start radiating my abdomen next week. With that said, I went into my presentation and soon I felt like the old Mr. Lawrence that they were used to.

I can tell you that my cracked open neck was definitely an attention getter. The people at the gym eventually stopped staring. The weights training went out of the window, and the stair climber was less than a minute, which cause an uneasy breathing. However, I continued my daily visit to the gym, and my workout regimen had been reduced to just walking around the track at an extremely slow pace. At school, it seemed to anger some of my colleagues because I would not use the elevator. It took at least two to three minutes to climb the stairs, and when I reach the top, I would always be gasping for breath. I remember Mrs. Daon, one of our government teachers, adamantly expressed, "Mr. Lawrence, please start using the elevator." Then there was one of older Earth Science teachers name Mrs. Wright, who is forever etched in my head because of one of her statements made during a parent/student/teacher conference. The young man had gone home and told his mother that Mrs. Wright was mean and ugly and did not like him personally. To say the least, the young man's mother was already steaming when she arrived. Once Mrs. Wright arrived at my office, she greeted the mother, took a seat, and said, "I know that I am a bear and I ain't much to look at either, but your son needs the structure that I am going to provide for him." With that said, everything else was uphill, and the conference was a success. Anyway, I thought that I would give you a snapshot of Mrs. Wright's candidness. One morning, Mrs.

Wright came by my office, peaked in, and said, "You look real bad, why don't you go home?" I replied, "I feel fine but thanks for your concern." She then proceeded around the loop straight to Mr. Morgan's office. The next thing I knew, Mr. Morgan was in my office saying, "Randy, Mrs. Wright said that you look terrible and should be sent home?" I then said to Mr. Morgan, my kids are here at school, my wife is in the streets, and there is no one at home, so at least if I fall out here, someone can dial 911! We both had a booming laugh. He returned to his office, and I continued my counseling duties.

The "cracked open neck look" seemed to linger longer than I expected. So let me share a few cracked open neck stories. My eldest brother Henry owns Lawrence Landscaping and employed sometimes people that needed a second chance. He gave his company a Christmas party at the Officer's club at Fort Story. Celinda and I attended. There I was with one of my collarless shirts and the eye catching cracked open neck. The food and music was divine, and I was just enjoying myself to the hilt. The gawking was at an all-time low, and I'm sure the dark atmosphere may have had something to do at that though. After loading up on diet coke and dancing in slow motion, I headed for the men's room to release some pressure building up in my bladder. Once I was there standing in front of the urinal, one of Henry's employees came up to the urinal next to mine's, whips it out, and then looks over at me and in a loud voice said, "Goddamn, what in the hell happen to your neck." I thought for moment here's my chance to get some sympathy, so I replied with that I had cancer and was receiving radiation treatments. He then expressed in his loud voice again, "Well you better tell your doctor to give some of that chemo shit! Cause that mother fucking radiation has burned the hell out you!" I was so overcome with laughter that I started coughing, which interrupted my stream of urine.

By mid-December, my snail's pace was even slower. It then started to hurt when I laughed, and singing was definitely a thing of the past. Oh God! Is this a test? I cannot do my most treasured actions, laughing and singing, which saturated my psyche. I knew that the challenge would be tough; however, I was not prepared to be stripped of the things that produced jubilance in my life. I thought this must be the test of my faith, and I was determined not to wavier. But then again I thought, can I live without laughing and singing? Well, singing I guess I could let go for a while, but the laughing would just have to hurt.

One Sunday morning, my extended family wanted to meet at the Golden Coral for brunch. This was something that we did periodically, descend on the Golden Coral and eat until we literally had to be rolled out of that place. So there we were getting ready for the morning feast. Celinda purchased matching shirts for us a few years ago, and she suggested that we wear them. The shirts had collars, so I left a few buttons open keep the material from rubbing up against the exposed neck area. Then Celinda looked at me and said, "You should really cover that up." I said but Dr. Walker said not to cover it up. She explained how it may disgust people at the restaurant, so I agreed to let her wrap my temporary cancer trademark. She did an excellent job wrapping it, and once I buttoned up my collar, no one would ever know that it was disgusting up there. Celinda, the boys, and I loaded into the Impala and off to Golden Coral for family fellowship and to satisfy our ravenous appetites. Once we arrived at the Golden Coral, my siblings and their kids and grandchildren started entering the establishment, filling the room with laughter and hugs and kisses. I had not seen my two brothers Henry and Page for a couple of weeks so they did not know about my neck condition. It's funny now, but when they both greeted me at different times of course, each one went in for the kill and grabbed me around the neck. Oh, the pain, with the cloth sinking deeply into my moist meaty neck. I just smiled and gave a big hug. Overall, the bunch encounter was a plus for my spirits. Unfortunately, I became angry with Celinda for convincing me to let her perform her unneeded wrapping. I made the mistake of telling her my feelings and asking if she were trying to delay my recovery time. This is when the shit hits the fan, so to speak. I saw and felt her Florence Nightingale support explode, and it was the inauguration of the emptiness that plagued our relationship. Shortly after that incident, Celinda and I were discussing our relationship when she expressed not really loving me anymore and would be moving out soon. She started sleeping in the guest room but still used our bedroom for hygiene things and getting dressed.

Chapter 5

Tallwood Coming to the Rescue

At school, the love and support was really beginning to pour into my life. So many acts of kindness and unconditional support from family, friends, faculty, students, and parents left me in tears of joy quite frequently. One day, Daddy and Mama B unexpectedly showed up at school with a floral arrangement that was absolutely beautiful, with a get well soon card attached. When they entered my office with the spirit-lifting vase, I burst into tears, and Mama B replied, "Oh Randy, please don't cry." Then Daddy said, "B! Let him cry if he wants too." What a rare moment for me to see a sensitive side to my father. Then there was Laura Jones, one of my alumni students who was currently attending Old Dominion University. She came by with a huge casserole meal. She put down the casserole, gave me a big hug, and said that she found out that I was meeting the cancer challenges and prepared something for me and the family so I would not have to cook that evening. Water works started uncontrollably, and my soul immediately filled up with gratitude. Oh don't let me forget the surprise from another one of my students, Jason Ingram. It was one morning about ten minutes before the bell when Jason entered my office and said, "I heard that you had a death in the family." I looked puzzled trying to figure out who had died that I couldn't remember. Then he placed a flannel shirt with something inside on my lap. The shirt began to move, and as I started to unwrap it, I discovered a puppy from heaven, and tears began to flow. I called Celinda to come to pick up the bundle of joy to take back home. The puppy was a mixed breed of chocolate Labrador and pit bull. We named her Coco. Lamarr and Jason were so happy to have a new dog around the house. Coco was so high strung, we should have named her loco. She was all over everyone and everything twenty-four seven, barking, licking, chewing, jumping, and running. What a completely different demeanor from our mild-mannered Poochie.

Life at Tallwood was my refuge. I could always count on the students or Mr. Morgan to make me laugh until it hurt literally. In addition, this haven provided me with a sense of purpose while slowly maneuvering through my cancer journey.

One morning, Mrs. Peggy Peebles, one of our assistant principals, came into my office and put hand on my shoulder and uttered, "Lord Randy, you need to come with me." I said, "What's up Peggy?" And she said, "It's Lamarr!" I said, "Oh my god! Is he hurt?" She shook her head no and said, "Come with me, he's in the principal's conference room." When she opened the door, Lamarr was seated at the conference table with his back facing me, and there was Mr. Morgan, the school police officer, and a couple more assistant principals seated and staring at me when I entered the room. I walked in bent down, put my arms around Lamarr, and said, "I don't know what you have done, but whatever it is, we will work through it together." Lamarr was working at the Activities Office downtown. He lifted a few adult activities passes and sold them to his friends for a dollar. At one of the home football games, one of our students presented the adult activity pass to gain free entry. When she was questioned about the origin of the pass, she became very evasive. When the police officer responded with this is stolen property and is punishable by completing some jail time. Lamarr Lawrence's name rolled off of her lips so eloquently. Again this could be another long story, so I will sum it up by saying that he ended up with ten days of out-of-school suspension, and Celinda and I had to go before the school board to have our son restated at Tallwood so that he could complete his senior year. There we were, sitting before a panel of three school board members. When it was time for me to speak on Lamarr's behalf, it felt like an hour had passed during my travel from the bench to the podium. Once I took my place at the podium, all I could do was ask for forgiveness. We all knew Mars was guilty; however, he was also very remorseful. Mr. Morgan's supporting recommendation for Lamarr to be restated at Tallwood was a major factor for the school board's decision to let him return to his home school. That's when I started thinking between Lamarr and Celinda, I just might not make it through this cancer journey.

We also ushered as a family at the Wells Theater in Norfolk. I signed the whole family up in 1993 as members of the Virginia Stage Association and received the family discount. There were at least six plays a season, and our family would choose one night to usher for each play. Our duties consisted of arriving an hour and a half early and stuffing play bills, and once the patrons arrived, we showed them to their seats and clean up the theater of trash before we left the building. Celinda and I usually covered the two left doors on the mezzanine section or took tickets at the front door, and Lamarr and Jason always covered the two doors upstairs to the balcony. Once the doors were closed, we were permitted to enter the theater and take an empty seat or in the mezzanine section with their high chairs behind the theater seats. This was a great family outing; we got to see all of the plays for free and became critics in the process. We were a great team. The drive home was filled with laughter about our comments about the plays. Also, standing and facing Celinda at the door and exchanging comments about the patrons was something special for me. She always looked so good. Little did I know then that "A Christmas Carol" would be the last play that we ushered together that December.

Christmas 1995 came quickly even though I was moving slowly. Celinda and I always collaborated in creating the family Christmas card to distribute to family and friends. Because I was in my mental and physical fried state, Celinda took on the project with input from me and the boys. She decided to create a newsletter, something that I really didn't want to send. I thought newsletters sucked because the ones that we received in the past seemed like opportunities for people to brag about all they have and all they have done. However, I must say this newsletter she created captured the essence of what the Lawrence's were experience during that moment. Here's her master piece.

LAWRENCE EXPERIENTIAL GAZETTE

1995 Overview
Vol. Vol. I No. Issue I
December 1995

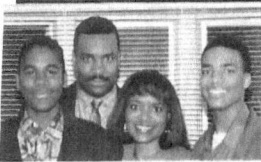

One Day at a Time

Everything's going to be alright.

Randy Lawrence

Having cancer does have it' s conveniences. It is most effective when you want to get rid of pesky sales people or if your desperate for a fail proof way to lose weight. Other than that, the cancer experience is painfully tiring and consistently bothersome. At the midway phase of my therapy I can honestly say the cancer is mentally and physically draining. But, I am an optimistic, God dependent, laughing soul that refuses to allow this intruder to still my joy.

What ever do you say to the person that has cancer? Well I've heard enough "everything's going to be alright" for two life times. And then there are the "I know someone with cancer" stories that don't really ease the mind. And how about the "you look great" comments. Some far more helpful gestures would be to offer a listening ear, ask what you can do to help, send an inspirational card, tell a really funny joke, include them in your prayers and don't ask them how it's going unless you really want to know.

CONTENTS

You really do learn from your mistakes.

Lamarr Lawrence, 17 years old

My folks have spent 17 years trying to teach me things like values, empathy, sensitivity, good judgement but it wasn't until I made a really dumb decision did I come to an understanding of what they'd been trying to instill in me. When you do something really stupid, I've learned that it can also impact on you family, friends and sometimes innocent people. My experiences this year have taught me that it is wise to think through a decision before making it and to anticipate the consequences of my choices.

Planning is also a way to avoid making haphazard decisions. I'm planning on going in the Marines and of course to get my Isuzu, Rodeo.

The flip side of this years craziness is that I've seen what family support and friendship is really about. Even though the people that care about you don't like some of the thing you do, they can forgive and still love you. I know about that because that's what happened to me.

Driving Mr. Lawrence

Jason Lawrence, 15 years old

I've gotten some great driving experience this year by driving my dad to his radiation treatments. Not only am I getting driving experience but my folks tell me that I've been a big help to them. I prefer to drive the 54 Chevy but I'm going to also learn to drive a stick shift.
This has been a busy school year, a devoted Bills year, and a steady growth year (I'm 6' 2" tall).

Schooled out.

Celinda Lawrence

Nursing school has been a painstaking experience and I don't know exactly why. Perhaps it's the over 40 perspective, the 10 pound school books, the test provoking anxiety.. Whatever the cause I'm schooled out.

This year has just flew by and there were so many things left undone. But the things that did get done were done well.

The big picture

by All of us.

When you look at a picture it is so easy to focus on the small minute flaws that you can loose sight of the essence of the picture in it's entirety. This year has had it unexpected twists , but the joy we've gotten through the Lord, our family, and friends has put things in their proper perspective. We've learned to take things one day at a time, enjoy the nightly rest that replenishes us, take nothing for granted and to strengthen our relationship with God. Thanks for being a part of our big picture. Keep the Lord's words close to your heart and mind .

Celinda's Slamming Sour Cream Pound Cake Recipe

by Celinda

3 cups all purpose flour
3 cups sugar
2 sticks butter
1/4 tsp. salt
1/4 tsp. baking soda
6 eggs
1 cup sour cream
1 tsp. vanilla
1 tsp. lemon

Cream margarine and sugar.
 Add one egg at a time.
 Beat well.
Fold in flour, fold in cream.
Add flavorings.
 Pour in large greased and floured tube pan.
 Bake 325 for 1 ½ hours.

Crumbs from the Counselor's Table

by Randy

Adolescence can be a tumultuous time in a young person's life, Not only are their hormones zapping their bodies into metamorphis but their minds are also undergoing adventurous and sometimes irrational thoughts. As a guy who interacts with teenagers on a daily basis, I have found the following tips to be very effective:

-Listening is an essential tool to apply with teens

-Allow periods of silence because time may be needed to collect one's thoughts

-Offer unconditional support by being there through the ups and the downs

-Delay passing judgement until explanations have been made.

-Apply punishments that fit the offense.

Finally, keep in mind that just as the terrible Two's, this time too will pass.

Rapping with Lamarr

by Lamarr

My folks are always asking me about rap music. They just don't understand why it appeals to so many people. Non rap lovers hear the music and all they can think of it is that it's about killing and drugs. What they don't realize is that rap is usually telling the truth about people's lives. If you listen clearly it tells you of hardships, deaths of friends and love ones and prison life. This is a reality for many people and for others it's unreal. Rappers are expressing themselves in

a different music form. Rap is just an option, it is not for everybody. That is the beauty of America, we have the right to choose from our options. I chose rap.

Sticking with the Bills

by Jason

The Buffalo Bills are the best team to ever play in the NFL. There are not any other tems in the NFL that have been to the Superbowl four consecutive times (I think). It does not matter who wins the Superbowl, the challenging achievement was making it into the Superbowl. One game should not account for a season's amount of hard work. These are simply the opinionated heartfelt words of a serious Bills fan.

AND WHATEVER YOU DO, WHETHER IN WORD OR DEED, DO IT ALL IN THE NAME OF THE LORD JESUS, GIVING THANKS TO GOD THE FATHER THROUGH HIM. COLOSSIANS 3:15-17

Blessed holidays to you. We have really enjoyed putting this newsletter together. We wanted to share ourselves with the folks we just don't get to see or hear from as often as we'd like.

That Christmas morning, we did the same yearly ritual, which consisted of opening the gifts and taking photographs to freeze the moments. The kids always appeared to be happy with whatever Santa left; however, by then they were very aware of the real Santa Claus. That Christmas, my in-laws invited us over for breakfast. So after the gift celebration by the Christmas tree, we went upstairs to dress for the occasion. Once everyone was dressed, we headed out the door, and Celinda and kids were in the car in a flash. I remember moving as fast I could, and while creeping, I noticed Celinda looking at me with disgust in her eyes. It took a couple of minutes for me to get into the car. I finally arrived at the car, opened the door very slowly, and sat in the front seat on the passenger side. Celinda's eyes met mine, and she uttered in an unpleasant tone, "Can you move any faster than that?" Unfortunately, I interpreted this jester of questioning as a tongue lashing and a strong indication that maybe I was just faking. I could feel the boys' eyes on my back; however, silence filled the interior of the automobile. I did not respond to her question. That discerning look and tone of questioning made me feel so less of a man. I could not believe how I had been Mr. Everything now reduced to Mr. Nobody.

Christmas Day was a dinner at Olivia and Ronald's home traditionally. Olivia was the only one of my siblings still living in Creeds, next door to the house where we were raised. The Dabneys had lots of space and always had a minimum of two big Christmas trees in a couple of rooms, with festive decorations all over the house inside out. Dinner was always excellent. Olivia and Ronald would collaborate on the cooking and made a meal that as they say would "make you slap your momma." Before dinner, we joined hands to make the circle of trust, and Daddy said the blessing. Then a line would form visiting the various areas where the mouth-watering entrees were placed. Olivia love to play games and has an inspirational way of motivating people to participate. So during and after dinner, there was always something to simulate the mind and break the ice, which normally leaves everyone in stitches. Then we would break out singing Christmas Carrols, with my Aunt Bertha on the piano and Cousin Tommy on the organ. Going home produced a nostalgic feeling of growing up in Creeds. We would usually walk up the lane and give greeting to my extended family, which always provide a stimulating conversation of old times between family members. I was unable to make the up the lane walk that year.

Chapter 6

Radiation Down Below Time

Twenty-four down and twenty to go, bring it on! Right after Christmas, I started the treatments to my abdomen and below. Up to that point, my weight had remained the same. My ride after radiation treatments still left me very sleepy, and Jason continued to drive us home safely every weekday. It wasn't until after about the fourth treatment that I began to feel different physically. I treated my cousin Anthony whom I hadn't seen in years to dinner at Apple Bee's on Lynnhaven Parkway. We were enjoying sharing the happenings in our lives and reminiscing about the past. I was eating their delicious Phil steak cheese sub when I became very nauseous. I immediately looked at Anthony, and he said, "You don't look so good." I respond I don't feel very well either, and then I rapidly jumped from the chair and sprinted toward the restroom at a speedy turtle's pace. Unfortunately, before I reached the restroom, I experience an upsurge from my stomach, which transformed into a distasteful, pungent smelling mush discharged from my mouth, gracing the carpet in the dining area. Thank God, it was only a small discharge before I managed to make it to the men's room and polluted the toilet bowl with a huge deposit of acid vomit. Once my stomach stop churning, I returned to the table with Anthony, displaying sad eyes expressing ambivalence about the dinner date ending so abruptly.

It was not long after the dinner date with Cousin Anthony that my love affair with food was put on hold. My desire to eat was significantly reduced. Then the thing that put me over the edge, Winky (my penis; by the way, they say it's normal for one's penis to have a name), took a sabbatical. You know what I am saying, no morning erections or any erections at all. I could not believe Winky's death from a man named Randy. I pretty much stayed in that Randy state physically and mentally for most of the day before that dolorous morning. I remember thinking what on earth can I play with now that will bring me even half the pleasure I used to experience with Winky in my hands? Oh Lord, I lost my appetite, it hurts to laugh, singing required work, and now Winky is dead, are there more lessons for me to learn, or are you preparing me for something bigger and better? I held on to the notion of bigger and better. In the beginning of this cancer ordeal, my doctors told me Hodgkin's disease was the best cancer to have if it is caught in stage one. You know, the Lord only gives me the best!

It wasn't long before the pounds started to disappear. Even though physically I felt like crap, image wise I felt fantastic because I was able to wear all the clothes I purchased when we lived in Berlin, Germany. Back in my 34-inch waistline pants, oh yeah! I was feeling like a stud even though I didn't have the stamina or a living Winky to perform in that capacity.

I was also starting to believe that Celinda was trying to get rid of me so that she could collect the $500,000 worth of life insurance. I made an appointment to see my lawyer, Attorney Koch, to express my concerns. Besides the being knocked off issue, I wanted to know what it would take to have Celinda removed from our home since she said that she was leaving and only moved to the guest bedroom. A series of things happened within a couple of weeks that spooked the hell out of me. One evening, I was on my way to Bally's driving the 54 and as I approached the intersection of Rosemont Road and Holland Road, the light turned red and I applied the brakes only to feel the brake pedal collapse rapidly on floor board and the 54 continued at a 45-miles-per-hour speed. There were a couple of cars stopped at the traffic light so I immediately turned to the right and drove into traffic taking off from the light. The cars yielded as I looked like a man in distress, and the 54 hit the center median on Holland Road, which slowed the car down tremendously, and the car coasted in the left-hand lane up a little when I made a left turn, crossed the two lanes, and into the parking lot of Brakes and Alignment Shop. Once I got control of my rapidly pounding heart, I had a word of praise for my Lord. I left the 54 in the parking lot and called that shop the next morning, and they made the repairs to the brakes.

Then one morning, I was driving to school when the rear axle on the 54 snapped; however, I managed to get the car off the road safe. The last incident put the icing on the cake. Most morning, I would always come around the 54 from the rear to enter the vehicle. This morning I'm not sure where my mind was but it must have been divine intervention, I walked around the front of the 54 only to find all of the nuts with exception of the lock nut screwed completely off and laying on pavement next to right front tire. The Lord knows I got scared and began questioning maybe someone is trying to put the lights out before I finish facing the cancer journey. After speaking with Attorney Koch, he assured me that the idea of Celinda trying to put my lights out permanently was ludicrous. Of course, I got a second opinion from Bob, one of my mechanics. In fact, all of the mechanics that worked on 54 assured me that the brakes and the axle breaking were not a part of any foul play. Somehow, with all that reassurance from everyone, I was still not convinced. The wheel nuts being unscrewed and laying on the pavement next to the tire were just an attempt of tire theft, or so I was led to believe.

One time, Mattie and Yvonne came for a visit during the middle of the week, and our plans were that they would pick me up at 11:00 a.m. from school and then we would drive up to the Pottery Factory in Williamsburg. They arrived at Tallwood right on time, and I could tell that Mattie was steaming about something. When we went out of the parking lot and headed toward Interstate 64, a flush of emotional conversation commenced. Mattie said, "This morning when Yvonne and I were getting ready to come over, the phone rang, and I picked it up and said hello. The voice on other end greeted me with 'Hello, baby, are we going to get together today?' I responded with 'Excuse me, to whom am I speaking with?' And he said, 'Come on, Celinda, this is Dennis.' Then I said, 'Dennis, this is not Celinda. I am Mattie, Randy's sister; however, I will make sure that Celinda gets this message.' Then there was silence on the phone, so I hung up." Let's just say that incident dominated the conversation on our way to Williamsburg. I really did not have the strength to get angry, besides I already had a strong suspicion that maybe Celinda was stepping out, but I did not have any concrete evidence. There were other things pointing to a possible affair. She told lots of good stories. She told me and the boys that she reserved a hotel room in Richmond for the weekend to have some study time. Since our communication was limited, I did not even bother to question that scenario. So by time I heard Mattie's telephone encounter with Dennis, I was much at peace with Celinda's actions; my main focus was healing. I did confront Celinda once with my suspicion of her having a man on the side. She responded, "What man would want me?" I immediately responded with don't you still have a pussy? Then there was silence, I guess you could call it our new favorite sound—the sound of silence. However, the thoughts of her hoping that my lights would stop burning or finding an accidental way to put my lights out continue to resurface periodically.

Finally, on January 24, 1996, came the last day of radiation. It was Olivia's birthday, so she accompanied me to last radiation session followed by a double celebration dinner at the Olive Garden. When I arrived home that afternoon, I was ecstatic to finally scrub the ink markings off of my body. The intoxicating smell of that ink markings faded from my body, and my nose enjoyed the smell of nothing. I always said that a clean smell is no smell. How refreshing to breathe air with no smell! My nose died and ascended to seventh heaven.

The radiation treatments were over, and Dr. Walker declared me cancer free and now officially in the big R for remission! I wasn't much of a man physically, but mentally I knew that recovery period for the burned insides would be a long road. I continued to go to the gym and started back on stair climb, maxing out the first time of twenty seconds before I was completely out of breath and gasping for air. I also realized how I missed sweating. What used to be somewhat embarrassing for me now was a desire to have back. After radiation treatments were done, visits to the cancer center to see Dr. Walker were schedule every three months, and in between those three months, I had appointments with Dr. Rao. On one of my visits to Dr. Rao, I asked for an explanation of what I was physically experiencing. Whenever I tried anything new or just tackle the stairs at a rapid pace, I would gasp for breath and my breathing become almost violent, which gave me the feeling of going into cardiac arrest. He explained that it was the scar tissue in my chest caused by the radiation, and when I do something physical, the scar tissue shifts and puts pressure on my lung, which manifests into restricted breathing. He told me to continue to exercise and things would get better, which I did. I even stepped up my exercise routine although periodically I would feel the pain. You know the deal, No pain, No gain!

Friday, February 9, Celinda and I attended Richard Wagner's "The Flying Dutchman" at the Harrison Opera House. I was burned up on the inside from the radiation treatments and quite frustrated from the noncommunication between Celinda and me. That date was one that will not go down in history for I was left with emptiness. Shortly after that cold day in February 1996, Celinda started to make me crazy. It was pure torture with her sleeping in the guest room and using the master bedroom for grooming. She paraded her sexy body over to our walk-in closet and used our bathroom to shower, which kept my mind in knots and slightly distorted. Even though Winky was on a sabbatical, watching her invade my space in an alluring fashion added to my sexual frustrations. One evening, the kids were downstairs watching TV, and Celinda was in the guest room studying after she had just finished one of her famous trips to our bedroom with closet and bathroom rituals. As I sat there on the bed, I became more and more obsessed with finding a way to ending this torture. I'm not sure when the idea or motivation occupied my mind, but I started taking her personal belongings out of the closet and walked to the guest room with her lying there on bed and threw her garments on the floor. Celinda had more than 200 garments hanging in the closet along with more than 100 pairs of shoes. This venture ended up lasting way past my bedtime, which was 8:30 p.m. After every trip carrying as much as I could fit in my arms, I was forced to take a two-minute break between each trip to catch my breath. No one said nor did anything to stop me in all my madness. I was determined not to stop until all of Celinda's personal belongs were out of what used to be our bedroom. I finally accomplished my mission after four and a half hours then immediately collapsed on the bed and slept like a dead man. The next day, everything went back to cancer normal, except no more Celinda in and out of the bedroom. At that time, I did not think that my actions were a little twisted, until one of my Tallwood parents, whom Lamarr was best friends with her daughter, came to see me at school. She said, "Are you getting along OK, and how are things at home?" I replied with my usual things are all good with me. Then she expressed a great concern because she heard that I had thrown all of Celinda's clothes and shoes out of the bedroom. You could have purchased me for a quarter. I told her that I was just on a little moving mission, besides I did not have the strength to throw anything and stressed to her how all items were placed in another room. I am not sure if that satisfied her curiosity, but I was finished with an explanation of my action. It was quite some time after that incident when Celinda and I actually exchanged a few words, she told me, "If you want me to move my things out of the bedroom, all you had to do was ask." I did not see anyone trying to help me with the big move on that day. Maybe her statement wasn't so accurate.

By mid-February 1996, my workout at Bally's on the stair climber had progressed from twenty seconds to five minutes. I was determined to get back to pumping that exercise machine for an hour. Every day, I added twenty seconds to my time on the stair climber and would finish with a walk around the track until the spirit could not move me anymore, which sometimes would only be about five minutes, totaling a whopping two times around one-eighth of one-mile track.

Also in mid-February, my biking buddy Keith asked if I had the stamina to participate in the multiple sclerosis (MS) 150 bike tour in June. The 150 MS bike tour was something I did every year since returning back home in December 1991. In fact, the first MS 150 bike I participated was in 1985. I won a Slid Lid helmet, which I still wear to this day, for being the second highest fund raiser. I turned to Keith on to the MS 150 bike tour, and he completed his first ride in June 1994. I took the challenge and asked Keith if he could raise the money because I did not have strength to solicit for donations. Keith recruited more of his male friends and relatives and established us a team, which he named the Hurt-in Hiney's. I dusted off my Fuju road bike and started training in slow motion on the weekends to prepare for this big event. Keith and a couple of other Hurt-in Hiney's would periodically on the weekend get together with me to ride. Most of the time, I would always lag behind and Keith would stay with me.

February also brought a nice snow buildup that covered the grass to perfection and left the roads drivable. The boys and I grabbed the two German shields that we purchased while living in Berlin, slowly jumped onto the Impala SS, and headed out to Mount Trashmore. Upon arriving at the entrance of Mount Trashmore, we were wide-eyed to see the number of people sliding down the mountain. I parked the car, and Lamarr and Jason jumped out with the shields, checked whether I would be OK, and were up the top of the mountain before I even made it to the bottom from the parking lot. I saw the look of pure exciting joy on their first trip. They suggested that I do it for the feeling was incredible. So I started my journey around Mount Trashmore to the concrete stairs that led to the top. Every two steps on what seemed to be an endless stairs, my heart would start beating rapidly and my breathing would increase almost to the state of hyperventilating. I would stop until I felt somewhat normal before continuing my climb. I know that Lamarr and Jason probably had been up and down at least ten times before I reached the top. Upon mastering the last step, my breathing was so profound and my heartbeat pounded so hard I felt like it was going to crack my rib cage and burst out of my chest. After an extended period of resting at the top, Lamarr gave me his shield. There at the top of Mount Trashmore, I positioned my body on the shield and made my victory descent. It was a few seconds of flying freedom as snow sprinkled on my face and blood rushed through my body spreading jubilance. Wow! What a feeling that I wanted so badly to feel those few seconds of ecstasy one more time. However, I knew in my heart that another climb like that my result in my demise. Jason took the shield and carried it back up, and he and Lamarr continued in the festivities. I watched my sons enjoy the snow like the days when we were in Berlin. There were all kinds of boards and household apparatuses being used to obtain that rush from a speedy ride down Mount Trashmore. We selected the guy using the hood of a car as the most unique mode of transportation, and boy was that thing leaving a snow jet stream of smoke on its descent. After we had been out there for about an hour and half, the Virginia Beach Police officers arrived on the scene and busted up the fun. They made everyone get off the mountain and exit the park and said what we were doing was extremely dangerous. So without delay, we rapidly exited the park and went with a new experience under our belts.

February 21, 1996, I woke up to a big surprise and had no one to share it with. What a moment and a great day to rejoice for Winky was standing tall and proud! I did not know what to do with my friend who had awakened from a dormant state. I do know that was my first sign of healing from radiation. I thought, does this mean the big "O" was a possibility? Needless to say, I really did not have time to experiment at that moment because I had to get ready for work. However, I did share my morning experience with Mr. Morgan and Gay, which generated a tremendous amount of laughter throughout the day. When I arrived home after work, my mind started to become entangled with frustration. I deliberated Celinda's current voluntary sleeping arrangement and what would the consequences be if I jump her bones right there in the guest room or took matters in my own hands. So I chose to take matters in my own hands. First things were feeling as natural as my actions in the past, until the big spit came, then it felt as if my heart was going to burst out of my chest with an uncontrollable breathing that nearly scared me to death. So I decided that maybe I was rushing things and should give Winky a break.

Friday, March 15, was opera time again, and Celinda said she did not plan to attend because she had some studying to do. I asked Patsy to accompany me to Gioacchino Rossini's most famous French opera buffa (comic opera). This was a good opera for Patsy to attend because it was fused with tragedy, comedy, lively music, and drama. Patsy also accompanied me to Tallwood's junior ring dance. It was the first time that Celinda had not attended that function with me. I'm sure there were questions in everyone's head when I introduced my sister on my arms. I got a few "Where is Mrs. Lawrence?" I said she had to work. We had a great time even though I could not throw down at the ring dance like in the past; cutting the rug in slow motion is not the most attractive thing to see. The junior ring dance and the senior prom was always something that Celinda used to attend with me. Our dating days were coming to an end, and I was slowly dying inside. This lady that I enjoyed spending time with was now becoming a source of my contention.

In mid-March, the time came for Tallwood High School's fourth annual Student Faculty Follies. The Guidance Department had a sterling reputation for stealing the show when it came to the faculty acts. Let me give you a little of the pervious performances of the Guidance Department.

In 1993, we dressed like the Village People. We came out in two's and danced to different drumbeats provided by Kevin, one of my students, and another one of my students, Andy, played the keyboard. Linda B as a construction worker and Sherry as a nurse came out together from the opposite side of the stage to a mambo beat, followed by Patsy as a doctor and Elsie a chef to a disco beat, and Donna as a student, who did a chart wheel, and Gay in a gangster attire, who did a Michael Jackson spin to a hip-hop beat. Cheryl, dressed as a college graduate, and I, dressed in my army dress blue evening uniform, entered last to a funky beat, and once we joined the ladies out front of the stage, we sang Tallwood Guidance, a song in which I rewrote the words to the Village People's "YMCA."

"Tallwood Guidance"

Students—if you're feeling low
I said students—there's a place to go
I said students—we'll boost your ego
We will help you be successful

Students—if you feel like a bum
I said students—there's no need to feel dumb
I said students—there's a place you should come
We will help you be successful

Chorus

You ought to go to—Tallwood Guidance
Just get a pass to—Tallwood Guidance
You'll be on the right track
You will never look back
And a scholar you will be

Students—if your grades are bad
I said students—when your parents are mad
I said students—and you're feeling bad
We can help you be successful

Students—if your future's a mess
I said students—you should come to the best
I said students—you'll be put to the test
We will help you be successful

(Repeat chorus)

Students—are listening to me
I said students—what do you want to be
I said students—come to guidance and see
We will help you be successful

Students—we are all here for you
I said students—what do you want to be

I said students—of what you should do
We will help you be successful

(Repeat chorus)

In 1994, I rewrote the words to "Jesus Can Work It Out." Kevin smoked the drums and Andy fire up the keyboard again. We were all dressed in choir robes, and at end of the song, we disrobed and was dressed in our Village People out fits from the previous year and sang the last verse of "Tallwood Guidance," while Mr. Morgan, dressed like Rick James wearing a Rick James wig, entered the stage gyrating and for the big finish ripped off his shirt. The audience took screaming and laughter to a whole new level. The Guidance Department had topped the year before.

"Guidance Can Work It Out"

> Chorus 1
2×   Guidance can work it out—if you let them
        Guidance can work it out—Guidance can work it out

That problem that I had	I had
I just couldn't seem to solve	To solve
I tried and I tried	I tried
Just to keep it calm	It calm
I stopped worrying about it	Bout it
I turned over to guidance—and they worked it out	
And I said Guidance	O-oh yea

Chorus 1

The pain that would not move	Wouldn't move
I cried in my classroom	Classroom
The pain that I bore	I bore
I wondered how much more	Much more

But turned it over to guidance	Guidance
I stopped worrying about it	Bout it
I gave over to Guidance—Any they worked it out	O-oh yea

Chorus 2

And I said Guidance	Guidance can work it out
If you let them	Guidance can work it out
Oh-oh Guidance	Guidance can work it out
If you let them	Guidance can work it out

Listen here—that habit that I had	I had
I just couldn't seem to break	To break
I tried and I tried	I tried
Thought it would be too late	Too late (kick)
Gave it over to Guidance	Guidance
I stopped worrying about it	Bout it
Gave it over to Guidance	Guidance
Gave it over to Guidance	Guidance
3× I stopped worrying about it	Bout it

3× I gave it over to guidance	Guidance

I stopped worrying about	Bout it
I gave it over to Guidance—and they worked it out	O-oh yea

And I said Guidance	Chorus 2 (slow)
Guidance can work it out	Work it out
While you're trying to figure it out	Work it out
Already worked it out	Work it out
How you going to pay your rent	Work it out

When all your money spent	Work it out
Little bit to buy some food	Work it out
Baby needs a pair of shoes	Work it out
Look you have a light bill due	Work it out
Even got a gas bill too	Work it out
Telephone disconnected	Work it out
Waiting for your next pay check	Work it out

| 4× Tell you what you ought do | Work it out |

Guidance will see you through	Work it out
Witness they will see you through	Work it out
I'm a witness they'll see you through	Work it out

Mary was being harassed	Work it out
By several students in her class	Work it out
She heard teasing in the hall	Work it out
She even heard things at the mall	Work it out
Mary was sad and blue	Work it out
She didn't know what to do	Work it out
She came to Tallwood Guidance	Work it out

| 3× Didn't they didn't they work out | Work it out (orig) |

Joe was taking Algebra I	Work it out
The class was just no fun	Work it out
Every problem he tried to do	Work it out
He just couldn't make it through	Work it out
Teacher came running to him	Work it out
With an E all in her eyes	Work it out
Joe you been working so long	Work it out
Stop before you cry	Work it out

Joe looked at the teacher	Work it out
Then looked up at the sky	Work it out
I don't have no doubt	Work it out
Guidance is going to work it out	Work it out
Didn't they didn't they work it out	Work it out
Oh just give over to Guidance—and they'll work it out	Oh-oh yea!

In 1995, I rewrote the words to "Here Comes the Hotstepper." Kevin graduated the year before and was attending Old Dominion University, so I met with him at his home to get the act together before we sprung it on the ladies and Mr. Morgan. Again the performance was outstanding. We dressed in hit-hop attire. Once we got into the song good, as I would sing each line about the ladies, the spotlight would shine on them as they would shake up a little bit, and the audience screamed with sheer delight. Mr. Morgan, sporting a dreadlock wig and a Rastafarian cap, made his grand entrance at the end of the song just as I started singing his verse. The crowd came unglued, and the students were screaming like crazy. Guidance had provided another surprising performance.

"Here Come the Hot Steppers"

Hit It Na Na Na

Chorus	
Here comes the hot steppers	Counselors
We're miracle workers	Counselors
If you have a problem	Counselors
We'll solve it like that	Counselors

No-no we don't lie
Yes, we'll let you cry
Anyone depressed can hear the counselors sing
A song that you don't know
But stick around and you'll know
The song we sing ah-oh ching-ching chang

Chorus

Extaordinary
Sometimes you'll stationary
Life seems to get so tough all the time
Act like you know—then go
Till you find—you don't know
Come talk to us—students every time

Chorus

Guidance ------------------------- Guidance

Breaking a bad habit
Can't seem to stop at it
The Guidance Staff yes we understand
We're daddy of mack daddies
It's a lesson learned maybe
Sin't no hommines gone play me
Top Guidance Staff

Chorus

No-no we don't lie
Yes we'll let you cry
Anyone depressed will hear the counselors sing
A song that you don't know
But stick around and you'll know
The song we sing ah-on ching-ching chang

Chorus

Guidance ------------------------- Guidance

Here comes Ms. Dailey	Counselor
She's the Guidance Director	Counselor
This is Cameron	Counselor
She'll test you like that	Counselor

Guidance ------------------------ Guidance

Here comes Ms. Thornberry	Counselor
She's the scholarship lady	Counselor
How about Ms. Foster	Counselor
She'll career you like that	Counselor
Here comes Ms. Beverly	Counselor
She'll orientate you	Counselor
How about Ms. Delaney	Counselor
Peer counselor you like that	Counselor
Here comes Ms. Rottet	Counselor
She'll greet you at the doorway	Counselor
Look at Ms. Barkley	Counselor
She'll schedule you like that	Counselor
Here comes Mr. Lawrence	Counselor
With a college recruiter	Counselor
Don't forget Guidance Helper	Counselor
They get you like that	Counselor

NA NA NA

Here comes Mr. Morgan	Principal
He's dynamite leader	Principal
Just catch in the hallway	Principal
He'll hug you like that	Principal

Now all that history just to lay the groundwork for the essences of the Student Faculty Follies1996, and why it was a challenge for me, having no physical stamina. However, I did manage to come up with an idea to perform a melody of songs with the guidance gang being artist impersonators—the Supremes, the Beatles, Elvis Presley, and James Brown. The guidance staff immediately embraced the idea and really got into developing their characters. Sherry Rottet, our registrar, got married and moved to Indiana at end of the previous school year. Judy Allison replaced her and was immediately indoctrinated into the guidance gang. Patsy, Donna, and Judy were the Supremes; Linda B, Elise, Cheryl, and Kathy were the Beatles; Gay was Elvis; and Mr. Morgan was the God Father of Soul, none other than James Brown. I would be Ed Sullivan introducing the "Really Big Show." I recorded the music, which consisted of twenty to twenty-five seconds of the various artists' songs in the abovementioned order in three sets. On opening night, we were in the Guidance Office making final adjustments to the costumes before hitting the stage. The Supremes were dressed in black sequence gowns and big black wigs. The Beatles were in black suits with skinny black ties, and Elvis was in a white jump suit with the collar standing erect around the neck. Gay even had her hair moussed up and standing tall on her head. Then there was Mr. Morgan in an off-white three-piece suit and an official James Brown wig. We were definitely ready to dazzle the crowd.

The curtains opened with me at the center stage, the Supremes to the far left, the Beatles to the far right, Elvis slightly behind me to the right, and James Brown positioned behind me slightly to the left. The stage was completely blacked out, with only the spotlight on as I announced the "Really Big Show." The audience cheered with each name that I introduced. The music started with "Stop in the Name of Love," and the spotlight went to the Supremes. The ladies let loose with the famous hand gestures. Then the spotlight went to the Beatles as they performed "I Want to Hold Your Hand." Then from there, the spotlight shinned on Elvis and then to James Brown. By time the third spotlight tour on James Brown was about to end, the audience gave a huge ah as Gay's husband, Don Dailey, drove his white 1957 Thunderbird convertible on the stage. I walked out on the stage, and the ladies helped me in the front seat, and all the artists gathered around the T-bird as the curtains slowly closed. The applause and screams were graciously accepted as the curtains reopened for our bows.

The Follies 1996 was my first performance in all of years of my marriage to Celinda that she did not attend. She was really wrapped up in her schoolwork. I began thinking this time I know it's for real. Her support had truly died, and I was becoming a faded memory.

At the end of March, Lamarr, Jason, and I spent a week in Sandusky, Ohio, during Spring Break. It was our first vacation without Celinda, so we really got the chance to have some guy time. We stopped in Baltimore, Maryland, for one night, and we celebrated Jason's sixteenth birthday with Mattie and Ralph. Mattie picked up some Popeye's Chicken and a nice cake. We smacked our lips on the chicken, sang the traditional birthday song, and Jason made a wish and blew out the candles. The next morning, we were off for our men's vacation. We divided up the driving, cruising all the way in the Impala SS, which was a growing moment for all of us. My sons were no longer boys but young men, and I was so proud that I was their father. Once we arrived, I could see that Lamarr and Jason were not impressed by our surroundings. We had just passed an Amusement Park that was closed for the winter, so I'm sure that they were wondering what in the world are going to do for a week. We checked in and shortly afterward proceeded to our home for a week. Our living accommodations consisted of a cabin-like duplex condo on stilts with a small set of stairs to climb to the front door a placed in very close proximity to Lake Eric. It was very spacious inside, with a great view of the lake and nice fire place. We did the usual, which consisted of visiting the nearest grocery story and purchasing enough food that would hopefully last for a week. It was bitterly cold, so most of our activities were indoors, with the exception of the motor car race track and a day trip to Detroit, Michigan, to visit the Rock and Roll Hall of Fame. I'm sure the motor cars were the highlight of Lamarr and Jason's first vacation with dad.

Chapter 7

Friends Visiting

Our first visitor from the past was Steve Wilberger, an army buddy. Steve was a mutual friend of Celinda and me. We met Steve in 1982 when I was stationed at Fort Davis on the Atlantic side of Panama. Steve's hair was completely gray, and he was beginning to lose some of his hair. Steve was then married to Heidi, and we thought that they were nice older couple in their early forties, until one day we had a company at the beach. Celinda, the kids, and I were playing in the sand when we saw Steve walking in our direction with just his swim trunks. I looked at Steve and then turned to Celinda and said man Steve has really taken good care of himself; he has the body of a young man. Boy, I sure hope that I can look like that when I'm in my forties. Of course, I had to inquire about Steve's secret to his youthful appearance, only for him to tell me that he was twenty-five and married to an older woman with kids not much younger than him. He said that he started prematurely turning gray in high school. Steve eventually divorced Heidi and met a beautiful lady from Africa name Monica when we were stationed in Europe. They fell in love and got married. Steve was then stationed at the Pentagon and living in Northern, Virginia, with Monica when he came down for a visit. Celinda moved back into the bedroom with me to make things look normal. Steve and I hung together most of his visit. It was fun to have a blast from the past and reminisce over old times in Panama. Celinda and Steve were in a play together, *The Owl and the Pussycat,* when we were living Panama. The show ran for a couple weeks at a theater on Fort Davis. They received great reviews, and I did not even get jealous when they had to kiss on the lips in a few scenes. Anyway, just before it was time for him leave, he said to me, "Are things OK between you and Celinda? Things do not feel right, and the guest bedroom feels lived in." I broke down and gave him my vision of the scoop, and he gave me the sad eyes and words of sorrow and encouragement has departed to return home.

The next visitor was my best friend Hugh B. Brown Jr. Hugh and I hit it off the first time we met when I first moved back home from Berlin, Germany, with three kids on December 13, 1991. It's kind of a neat story. Celinda and I separated while we were living in Berlin. I think our separation had to do with me being diagnosed with diabetes in September 1990. I am sure that diabetes made changes in my character that did not set well with Celinda. I really don't know why she left, but anyway, we had been separated about year and the kids lived with me. I know you're probably wondering how we went from having two sons, Lamarr and Jason, to three kids. Celinda and I adopted a little five-year-old girl name Stephanie in December 1987 while I was stationed at Fort Stewart, located in good old Hinesville, Georgia. Stephanie lived with us for five years before she returned to live with her foster mother Sandra Habersham, who live in Swainsboro, Georgia. (The Tales of Stephanie could be a title to the book.) OK, I got off track again; let's get back to my meeting with Hugh B. My cousin Renae invited me to one of his friend's New Year's party to meet some ladies because I was technically a single man with children. At the party, Renae introduced me left and right to women, and I was dancing like a crazy man. Then my Cousin Rose (Renae's sister) introduced me to Hugh, and we started talking and dancing with the ladies. Then we discovered we had common interest—bicycling. So we made a date to go riding. I would tease Renae from time to time on how she invited me to a party to meet some women for a possible mate and I left with a man.

Hugh moved to Durham/Raleigh area of North Carolina to secure a greater income in his career field of advertisement, shortly after Celinda returned from Berlin, and we got back together. Hugh was a really good listener, and I love him for listening to all of my Celinda stories and helping me to pull it back together whenever I would have Celinda breakdown in public. Anyway, Hugh came one weekend. We rode the bikes and dined out, and as usual, he became my emotional dumping ground. He left, and Celinda and I went back to silence once again.

My third visitor during this time was Deborah Jones. Deborah and I met in Berlin, Germany, while we were pursuing a master's degree counseling through Boston University's overseas program. Deborah and I had an instant mutual attraction to one another, so we immediately became study mates, and she was my partner during our hypnosis class with Dr. Susan McGinnes. Deborah and I really developed eternal bonding relationship. We always talked about getting counseling licenses and doctoral degrees, move to back to my home in Virginia Beach, and open a counseling practice and call it "Beach Therapy." She was not only intelligent, attractive, sexy, loving, caring, and great with my kids but also a cyclist, so together we rode all over Berlin. She always had a way of making me feel even better when I was already good to start with. She was a true friend for me and was a listening ear when I would experience a Celinda emotional breakdown in Europe.

Deborah actually received a counseling license and was currently enrolled at the University of Texas obtaining a PhD during my cancer days. After receiving our famous Christmas Newsletter, she contacted me immediately and made plans to spend a week with me in April. April came, and Celinda moved back to our bed (which we used for sleeping only), and Deborah used the guest room. Deborah had only been visiting one day, and on the second day, the hair started to grow back on my chest. She accompanied me to two of Jason's basketball games since Celinda did not want to attend either game. In addition, Deborah joined me on Sunday, April 25, to see Rodgers & Hammerstein's Operatic Musical "Carousel." I remember feeling lots of anxiety about being with a white woman. I felt like so many people were staring, which manifested into ambivalence knowing that if anyone had started something, I did not have the strength to protect us. Of course now I know it was all in my burned up lower brain. We planned a trip during that week and took a drive up to Baltimore in the 54 and spend a few days with my sister Mattie and her husband Ralph. Wednesday rolled around, and Deborah and I hit road with the 54. We had been riding an hour along Interstate 64 singing to Al Green's CD when I noticed the temperature gage, indicating that the car was running hot. I pull off at the next exit, and we jumped out and popped the hood, only to see steams escaping the radiator and a broken fan belt. There was nothing in site except some prisoners working on the road. We inquired from the prison guard of anything close by. He told us that there was a Kmart about a mile up the road. Deborah and I started our long and slow walk in the direction of Kmart. The prisoners where disbursed all along the highway, and their eyes were feasting on Deborah's assets. As we progressed down the highway, Deborah greeted and flashed a flirtatious grin to all the workers along what seemed like an endless path, which generated a spark of excitement in their eyes. That was a long and hot way to Kmart, but we finally reached this destination intact. We stepped into the automotive section calmly in search of the right replacement fan belt, being the one we had was broken and the electrical system of the 54 had been upgraded from generator to and alternator. We matched things up to the best of our ability and started that long and hot journey back to the car, with Deborah repeating her actions with the men on the highway. Once we got back to the 54, I went into my mechanic mode and discovered that the fan belt was too large. The correct size needed to be smaller than the one resting in the palms of my hands. My energy level would not permit a repeat trip to Kmart. Deborah saw my exhausted look/demeanor and happily volunteered to return to Kmart. Repeating her ritual with guys on the road, she returned with the correct belt in very little amount of time. Together, we installed the new fan belt and were off to the sounds of Al Green one more time.

Once we arrived in Baltimore, Mattie rolled out a red carpet just like she always did whenever I would visit. Deborah and I toured the parts of the downtown and just relished in the mellifluous moments of spending time together. The day before our scheduled time to return to Virginia Beach, we went out on the curb to find that the 54 had a serious malfunction. I ended up having the 54 towed to an auto repair shop that Ralph recommended. Unfortunately, because of the 54's age, it was going to take a couple of days to secure replacement parts. Things did not look good for the 54 joining the cars in traffic for our return trip. We had to get back, so Mattie offered the use of her red Chevrolet IROC Camaro. We said our good-byes the next morning and fired up the Camaro and hit Interstate 695 in a flash. Deborah and I were smoking that Camaro on Interstate 95, singing to the tunes on the radio. Just outside of Woodbridge, Virginia, the left rear tire blew out, and I applied the brakes gently to slow that baby down. After reaching a safe speed, I pulled into the center median on the road. Despite my grand attempt to exit the vehicle, I could barely physically make that happen. By the time I was standing erect by the car door, Deborah looked over at me and said, "I will change the tire." What delight for my the eyes when she rapidly took the keys out of the ignition, opened the trunk, removed the jack and the spare tire, loosened the nuts, jacked up the car, switched the tires, tightened the bolts on the rims, and jacked the car through the flat in the trunk all in less ten minutes. I knew she was good but had no idea she was that good! Soon the week of laughter and just feeling good was over, and Deborah returned to Texas. She left me feeling like a man once again, not to mention I actually had a small patch of hair sprouting out of my chest.

Chapter 8

Lamarr and Celinda Exit

When the senior prom time came around, Lamarr asked me not to attend, so I respected his request and did not go. That was the first time I missed Tallwood's senior prom.

In mid-May, my cousin Renae sponsored an annual birthday softball game. The boys and I always attended and really enjoyed playing softball. Renae was hot to trot. She had a few close girlfriends, and guys would come from all over to play. Renae has the right stuff to always attract the opposite sex. Renae would always choose me to be on her team, and I would be her pitcher. This time because of my limited physical abilities, I played the back catcher position. Also when our team was up to bat, I was assigned a designated run when it was my turn. Boy did that game take a lot out of me! Especially when a male runner leaving third base at record speed approaching the home plate and the just thrown ball from the short stop position made its way into my glove at that moment, the runner plowed into me with a velocity of a Mack truck and my body literally took flight and I landed on my back in a somewhat conscious state. Everyone rallied around me, and if you could have seen the Bette Davis stare Renae gave to the runner, it was a priceless moment. I was still intact and was able let out a healthy chuckle, and everyone hovered over my windless torso, immediately dropped the "kill the runner attitude," and quickly adopted the oh-my-god-is-he-OK expressions.

The last of May, Jason was inducted to the National Honor Society. The ceremony brought tremendous joy to my heart. All of my family and Celinda's family that lived locally came out to the huge event. Jason and Lamarr were both onstage that evening for Lamarr was a part of the program. He delivered one grandiose monologue. After the ceremony, we all gathered in the common area of Tallwood for a family photo. It was the first time in months when I did feel some tension between Celinda and me. It was also the time when Daddy's early stages of Alzheimer's disease were becoming very evident. Daddy kept wondering off from the group, and Celinda would always go to him and slowly bring him back in the fold.

I was getting around a little faster; however, June came rapidly, and the MS 150 Bike Tour was the first weekend. Keith picked me up early Saturday morning and made an easy trip to the Suffolk Airport. Once there, Keith registered the team, distributed the "Hurt-in Hiney's" T-shirts and contents in the registration package, and gave us an introduction plus a motivational speech. The MS 150 consisted of a 75-mile route from the Airport in Suffolk, Virginia, to Chowan College in Murfreesboro, North Carolina, on Saturday, then on Sunday, the return route was a completely different 75-mile route from Chowan College back to the airport in Suffolk. With the route in hands, we mounted our bikes and hit the pavement. I tried to keep up with pack, but it's very long (less than five minutes) before eating dust from the other cyclist. Keith tried to hang back with me, but I insisted that he do his thing and that would I see him once I made it to Chowan College. So finally, after multiple prompts from Keith, he broke away. In a flash, Keith was out of sight. The ride was not difficult for me; it was just real slow. In the past, I could easily ride seventy-five miles in four hours and always finished in the top ten percent of the cyclist. This time, it was a different story for it took me eight hours to complete the first seventy-five miles on Saturday. Sunday, was a kicker though for it took me almost nine hours to complete that last 75 miles. However, I was the only "Hurt-in Hiney's" team member to compete the entire 150 miles. My "Hurt-in Hiney's" riding buddies were dropping like flies for various reasons and jumping on the sag wagon to be transported by a pickup truck back to the airport. Even Keith bit the dust! I was one of last people to finish, witnessing a few vehicles left parked at the airport. Most of the cyclist had returned to the airport, enjoyed fellowship with music, food, and drinks, and had departed the premises. When I finally reached the gates of the airport, there were a few greeters there cheering me on! I could not believe I had completed 150 miles for two days and still not have a drop of sweat seep from my skin. However, what a thrill of victory that rushed through my veins knowing that I was really on the road to recovery.

I had one hundred seniors, including Lamarr, in my case load at Tallwood of the 410 graduating in June 1996. I managed to meet their needs and complete my responsibilities in a guidance counselor capacity, even though it was in a slow motion physical state. Writing letters of recommendations and preparing college applications for the students dominated my world of work. However, the interaction with my students created a feeling of wild anticipation over graduation. My eldest was graduating and had already been sworn in by the Marine Corps to leave on July 15 for Boot Camp. Graduation day came, and I handed each diploma to all of my students. After the ceremony, Celinda and Jason joined Lamarr and me outside of the Pavilion to snap a few pictures. That moment was bittersweet. I was overcome with joy about Lamarr graduating and totally frustrated with Celinda. We were still occupying the same house and shared zero communication. Later that day, I worked up the nerve to ask her when she was leaving. She said that she would not leave without a separation agreement. I thought to myself you have walked out over the last eighteen years three times and not once did you even use having a separation agreement a stipulation to exit the home. In fact, when we were living in Berlin, Germany, she exited the house empty handed, and I was required to get a separation agreement once I knew the kids and I were returning to the United States. I knew then it was time take action. I was sick of sharing the house with what I considered a cold and uncaring partner. I immediately made an appointment with Attorney Koch, and he drew a separation agreement at no charge. I brought it home for Celinda to review and sign. She refused and said that her lawyer will draw up a separation agreement.

The week after Lamarr's graduation, Lamarr, Jason, and I headed for Orlando for a two-week vacation. We stayed in Westgate Villas in Kissimmee, Florida. Celinda and I had purchased two timeshare back in June 1985. So I exchanged both timeshare weeks so that we could stay in one place for two weeks. The boys visited Disney World, Universal Studios, and other attractions there in Orlando. On the middle of Friday of our stay in Florida, Lamarr and Jason drove me to the airport in Orlando. I flew to Shreveport, Louisiana, to meet Deborah, Veronica (Deborah's roommate), Veto (a guy Deborah was dating, Bob Reshand (Deborah and I knew Bob from Boston University, we all had classes together in Europe), and a

sergeant friend of Bob whose name escapes my mind. Deborah reserved a
room at a hotel equivalent to the Quality Inn. On Friday night, we went
to a couple of clubs, and it was nice hanging out with Deborah, Bob, and
their friends. Soon we returned to the hotel to turn in for the night. There
two queen size beds in the room. Deborah and Veronica shared one bed,
Veto and I the other bed, and Bob and his friend slept on the floor. After
sleeping alone for the last six months, one night of sharing a bed with Veto
was no picnic. He moved quite a bit, and I was not used to sleeping with
someone breathing on your back. The next morning, I was happy to cough
up additional funds that had not been budgeted for this weekend excursion
to reserve a room of my own. I immediately checked into my room, and
it was long before Deborah came over to seek answers for my decision to
move out. I explained the issues I was experiencing and told her all was
well. After spending a day exploring with the crew, I slept like a baby. I had
a great time with Deborah and Bob, rehashing the past and speculating
about the future. The whole crew was attentive and did not make a big deal
about me moving slowly. Sunday morning, Veto drove me to the airport,
and I arrived back in Orlando. There, I was greeted with two large smiles
from Lamarr and Jason, waiting patiently to pick me up. I knew we have
raised two wonderful young men when I returned to the condo, and it was
the same as the way I left it. The last week went by so fast that my head was
spinning, and in a flash we hit Interstate 95 North returning home, which
produced a feeling of unrest for me. I told Olivia if Celinda was living there
that I was going to make some kind of preparation to move out myself. I
immensely desired that she was gone when we return home. To my dismay,
home girl was still lingering at home. I felt a severe depression coming
on. All this time, I was able to keep a positive attitude. Now there I was,
making a progress healing but slowly deteriorating mentally.

When we returned from vacation, I had my first public singing
engagement since the radiation treatments. Mrs. Butler, a math teacher
from Tallwood, asked me to sing at her sister's wedding. She heard about the
great job I did at Mrs. Fulford's daughter's wedding the previous year. They
requested that I sing the same song "I Believe in You and Me," the Four
Tops version. I met their church organist a few days before the wedding and
fire up the fried vocal cords. I knew at that moment that belting out a note
and holding that note for thirty seconds had vanished from my singing
abilities. What used to be so easy and natural now required concentration
and extra effort. On the day of the wedding, I was stationed up in the choir

stand with the organist. When it was time for my song, I stood up and put my heart in the song, and emotions ramped up as a few tears streamed down my face. After I finished singing, the organist looked at me, smiled, nodded, giving a stamp of approval. At end of the ceremony, I was told that I sang one soul-stirring rendition of "I Believe in You and Me." What joy filled my soul for God had given me my voice back. What a blessing!

On July 15, Lamarr left for Camp LeJune for basic training, and on the late afternoon of July 17 (Celinda's birthday), Celinda presented me with a separation agreement that she paid $300 to have drawn up by her lawyer. I was mentally beat down. I found a notary public, signed it without reading the document, although I told the notary public that I did, and gave it back to Celinda. She left the premises, vacated, moved her shit out of the house! Financially, Celinda only had two credit cards that had her name on them only and the car payment for the Impala SS. This reduced the monthly bill of $6,000 a whopping $850. This was not a major concern for me though. All I can remember doing was breaking into a holy dance! The weight was finally lifted, and I felt a renewed strength. That night, I slept in total peace and in a praise mode. I found later that she moved in with her parents and the separation agreement I signed said the same thing as the one Attorney Koch prepared for me. One day, I might understand the madness behind wanting to spend money on separation agreement. Also, this time I knew this was for real, for during the other separation between Celinda and I, the communication remained intact and sometimes the good physical loving too! During our eighteen years of marriage, this was Celinda's fourth time leaving the nest. With that said, now would be a good time to provide a brief history of the first time I met Celinda and her other three silent dramatic departures.

Chapter 9

Love at First Sight/Rocky but Spicy

In February 1975, a mutual friend, Jennifer Hightower, introduced Celinda and I to each other in the library at Norfolk State College. There she was sitting at a table wearing a nice simple little blouse with a pair of fitting jeans. When I looked into her beautiful large brown eyes, there was an instant connection for me, and from that moment, I could not get that lady out of my head. It was love at first sight! I did everything I could think to shake this new fantastic feeling, but to no avail, and the feeling just intensified. The next day, I searched the campus for the young sexy lady to confess my true love. I spotted her on the campus wearing a beige knit dress, accenting her booty from heaven, and a pair of high heels headed toward the library. Watching her walk for that brief moment sent my desires through the roof. I caught up with her, and during our elevator ride up to the third floor in the library, I confessed on the spot my true love for her. Of course, her response was not positive, and she strongly suggested that I had a few screws loose. However, all through the pouring of my hearting out to Celinda, I managed to convince her to go out with me just once. Being in her presence generated a level of excitement that was new to me. This new experienced feeling just made me glow all over. Knowing that I was soon going to have the opportunity to share some time with this baby doll made it difficult for me to concentrate on anything else going on in my life. The excitement and anticipation of having a date with a raving beauty nearly caused a physical explosion.

Our first date was at the Chrysler Museum in Norfolk. When I arrived at Celinda's family home located at the Princess Anne Plaza section of

Virginia Beach, it was raining like crazy. I knocked on the door, and her younger sister Janice let me in and said that Celinda would be ready in a few minutes. Once Celinda entered the living room where I was seated, she expressed discontinuing the date because of the adverse weather conditions. I said to her if you go out with me now, I promise you that you will not get wet. This is a true story as God is my witness. The moment we got ready to step out of Celinda's front door, the rain stopped. Once got into my 1973 Nova Hatchback (three-speed standard stick shift with a 307 V8 engine) and hit the Interstate 264, the rain started again. The moment we arrived in the parking lot of the Chrysler Museum, the rain stopped. Once we were in the museum viewing the exhibits and exchanging truly stimulating conversation, the rain came down in buckets. During the walk through the exhibits in the museum, I could not keep my eyes off Miss Celinda for she was equally as intelligent as her captivating beauty. God I wanted her to be a part of my life so badly. After we finished the culturally simulating atmosphere at the museum, the moment we headed for the car, it stopped raining. We got back in to the Nova and took the Interstate 264 again en route to the Virginian Steak House on Laskin Road in Virginia Beach. You know the story; it stopped raining when we pulled up into the parking lot of the Virginian Steak House. All through the consumption of our delicious meal and thought-provoking conversation, cats and dogs fell out of the sky, hitting the restaurants roof and adding a positive sound to what was already one intoxicating ambiance. The moment I paid the check and we set to the door to exit the building toward the parking lot, the rain stopped again. It was only a ten-minute ride to Celinda's home from Laskin Road, and believe or not, it rained until I pulled up in their driveway and escorted Celinda to her front door. Once she was in the house, it rained again and I got wet going to the car, and then I knew that it was true love. This was an inception of my days writing poems to the love of my life.

Written February 1975

I'm sorry I made you late to class
But that moment with you I wanted to last
To make you understand the words I say
Are true and I hope you'll believe them today
My feelings are something that can't be shoved aside
I want to share them with you so don't runaway or hide
I know you think I'm crazy or playing a game

But without you Celinda, I'm a face without a name
Celinda please tell me that you understand
For that small expression will make me your man
Even if you say, your love for me is in vain
I'll continue loving you just the same
So while lying here searching for myself in this world
Asking and praying that you will be my girl
To give and share your gracious beauty with me
Because I love you Celinda, and I want you to love me

Celinda

Celinda I am writing this poem just for you
To let you know how much I will do
To keep our love from drifting apart
For the thought of that breaks my heart
I know you think that I'm playing a game
But my love grows stronger for you just the same
You say there's no time in your life for me
But you and me together Celinda is the way it should be
My love for you I can't explain
But if you don't share your love with me I'll go insane
I love you and you know it, written on all the ceilings
So, Celinda please give in and stop fighting your feelings
You have extraordinary beauty and you know that's true
For without your existence the sky wouldn't be blue
Your friendly face and charming personality
Sends me spinning in space searching for reality
The radiance of your immaculate heart
Makes my body disassemble and fall apart
Celinda why don't you love me and stop acting so cold
For just a minute portion of your love will restore my soul
So Celinda, remember these feelings that I have expressed
And our relationship together will always be the best

Love always, Randy

Beautiful Lady

There is a lady named Celinda, I love so much
With skin soft as velvet, that's exciting to touch
A cute little nose and big brown eyes that I love to see
An effulgent smile with an expression of love for me
A sophisticated lady who's beautiful in everyway
The lady of my dreams, my sunshine in everyday
The lady who speaks and mind burns with fire
A lady when she walks, my heart agitates with desire
Celinda I love you that's all I'm trying to convey
I want and need you in a very special way
You're the lady that brings immense joy into my life
Yes you, beautiful Celinda my wonderful wife

Love Forever, Randy

Over the years, our relationship was rocky but spicy. We seemed to always have heated verbal altercation, which always ended with Celinda not wanting to see or speak to me again. Then one early summer day, I was riding with my brother Page who was driving one of my father's tractor trailer truck hauling a load to North Carolina. We were discussing my break up with Celinda and how much I still loved and desired her. Page said to me, "You are a Lawrence, and if you want that woman, go and get that woman." In July 1977, I brought Celinda an engagement ring, got down on my knees and proposed to her. She accepted, and a week later gave the ring back to me and said she did not want to see me ever again. In December 1977, guess who came back into my life? It was all peaches and cream, and we even finally consummated the relationship in my apartment at 721 Prince Arthur Court, in Virginia Beach. Talking about taking the relationship to a higher level. Man I was crazy in love. In January 1978, Celinda and I had a divergence, which resulted in a termination of our relationship one more time. To this day, I cannot tell you the causes of any of our break ups. I guess I was living in a fantasy world. After Celinda made her silent dramatic exit this time, I was broken hearted and decided I needed a change of climate—something wild and exciting to fill the love void. So I joined the army in March 1978 on the delayed entry program. My family was horrified; my boss at the Norfolk Adult Activity Center submerged my head into the bathroom sink filled with water and called me a black fool. My brother Henry, then Army Captain Lawrence, informed me of the huge mistake I was making for joining as an enlisted member, especially with already having a bachelor of science in accounting degree from Norfolk State College. I simply forgot the ridicule for my decision was incorrigible. I had to get out of the city.

In April, Celinda returned with the news of being four months pregnant and dolorous because of her preparation for medical school. She said that she was going to have the baby and her mother was going to care for the baby while she attended medical school. I told her that I want my half and was not in agreement with her mother raising our child. I unloaded the news of my army commitment and proposed to Celinda that night. I told Celinda that if she married me, Uncle Sam would pay for the birth of our child and she could take off after giving birth if she desired. She was pretty adamant about not loving me; however, I told her that I had enough love for the both of us. I also told Celinda that I had already promised my best girlfriend (since the eighth grade) Jackie Ellis that I would be her date at the school where she taught senior prom. We married on Friday, April 14, 1978, for all the wrong reasons at the marriage commissioner's home in Virginia Beach with my friend Joe Greene as a witness. That evening, I went to my second job in the shoe department of Leggett's Department Store at the Military Circle Mall in Norfolk. When I returned from work, Celinda informed me that my girlfriend Gwen Holloway (Gwen was my girlfriend from the eighth grade until I was a sophomore in college) called to congratulate me on getting married tomorrow. Unfortunately, I had told my family and friends that I was getting married that Saturday; however, Celinda insisted that we marry the day before because she did not want family members to attend.

Twelve days after we got married, I resigned from both jobs. Celinda resigned from the Norfolk General Hospital, where she was employed as a respiratory therapist thirty days prior to my entering the army. I went to the prom with Jackie, and we had a blast as usual. My report day for the army was on July 25, 1978, so the last thirty days, Celinda and I spent lots of time in bed together fine tuning our love making. After that, the mellifluous days Celinda and I shared together were imponderable, and the essence of our relationship was conceived.

Once in basic training, we corresponded daily through mail. The letters I received from Celinda during that period were filled with undying passion. On October 15, 1978, we were blessed with a seven-pound, eight-ounce baby boy, whom we named Lamarr Scott Lawrence. I got the name from the soldier who slept next to me in basic training at Fort Leonardwood, Missouri, named James Lamarr. Lamarr was born when I was attending finance school at Fort Benjamin Harrison in Indianapolis, Indiana. I remember so clearly when I first traveled home to see my son. I flew into Norfolk Airport, and once I got off the plane, I spotted Celinda dressed in a bronze form-fitting cowl neck dress, and right beside her black pumps supporting those well-defined long brown legs was a Bobby Mack baby seat with none other than Lamarr. We embraced, and tears ran uncontrollably down my face. I picked up my son, and the love poured out of my soul into this new creation of God. What a weekend (boot knotting galore). I returned to finance school, completed the training, and then I was off to my first duty station. In November that same year, I moved my new family to Fort Campbell, Kentucky, and rented a trailer at Clarksville, Tennessee. I was in December 1978 that Celinda uttered the words I love you. Joy and happiness entered and filled my soul. I thought this just might work out.

OK, here goes the rocky but spicy separations. Jason Wells Lawrence, our second son, was born on March 29, 1980, weighing in at five pounds and fourteen ounces, at Martin Army Hospital in Fort Benning, Georgia, while I was completing the Infantry Officer Basic Course (IOBC). I completed OCS at Fort Benning in January 1980 and was commissioned as a second lieutenant prior to attending IOBC. Upon completing the IOBC, we moved to Fort Eustis, Virginia, in May 1980. We lived on post for about a year until we purchased our first home, a three-bedroom one-bath ranch-style house located at 146 Merle Drive in Newport News, Virginia. Celinda was working odd hours with dialysis patients, and I was working at the Army Training Board. I was doing all of cooking, housework, and caring for Lamarr and Jason, which included taking and picking them up from day care. Celinda worked a lot but always manage to keep herself looking very sexy. I just could get enough of looking and being with her, until I just got tired of all of the extra duties plus picking up behind her. Did I tell you that I was anal retentive during that period of my life? Anyway, I stopped making love to Celinda, and fourteen days later she moved out. And you'll never believe who she moved in with until she got her own apartment—my best friend Jackie! Can you believe that? All I can say is that Jackie is really a good friend because she did not left herself get caught up in all of our shit.

Once Celinda moved out, I had a hard time making the $650 mortgage payment on a second lieutenant's salary. I solicited help from a roommate-finding service to find a roommate to help me with paying the mortgage. They immediately sent me a young man whose apartment building caught on fire and his girlfriend died in the fire. He was nice and all; however, I thought to myself that the boys and I did not need a depressed person living with us especially now, with them still adjusting to the absence of their mother. So I contacted Celinda since by that time she had moved out of Jackie's place and into her own two-bedroom apartment. I convinced Celinda to let the guy live with her and she could give his rent money to me so I could pay the mortgage. That worked out just find. Then I received orders to Panama, Celinda and I reunited. We moved to Panama and had a great life for we had a few live-in housekeepers the whole time we lived there.

The second separation came when we were living in Berlin, Germany. We adopted Stephanie in December 1987 when I was stationed at Fort Stewart, Georgia. We lived in Hinesville, Georgia, on an acre of land in a nice L-shaped white ranch house. Celinda was working crazy hours as a respiratory therapist in a hospital in Savannah, Georgia, which was at least a ninety-minute commute one way. So again I did the majority of managing the household. She had a burning desire to adopt a child to get a chance at improving what she thought she lacked in motherhood skills. I finally agreed to this quest. We attended adoptive parenting classes, and they matched us with Stephanie. Stephanie was born on August 28, 1982. She had been passed around from her biological mother, to her grandfather, and to foster care. It was not long before I received orders for another overseas tour. On September 1, 1988, we moved to Berlin, Germany, and left Poochie with Olivia and Ronald.

Once we got settled in Berlin, Celinda continued to pour all of her love and affection in being the best mother to the boys and especially to Stephanie. Unfortunately, the more Celinda did in loving Stephanie, the worst Stephanie would act toward her. Stephanie had a candid way of letting you know when she did not care for you. She verbalized very clear messages of her strong dislike when it came to Celinda and Lamarr. She merely tolerated Jason and me. Then on September 1, 1990, I was always thirsty, urinating every hour, fatigued, and had severe vision loss. I went to the military hospital and was diagnosed with diabetes, which is another book. Anyway, with diabetics, one must follow a restricted diet, which requires that sugar intake be significantly reduced to almost none at all. Remember, I stated earlier that Celinda had become quite the baker, and I was no stranger when it came to consuming her morsels of delight on a daily basis. Well, during the end of September 1990, she flew the coop for second time and moved into my friend Deborah Jones's flat. Deborah was living with her boyfriend, Kause, in his flat in the same building that he owned. So again my darling Celinda used one of my friends to help her escape her frustration in our relationship. Just before Christmas, that same year, she came back home, and reason for leaving this time was that she felt insignificant when she was unable to prepare pastries to satisfy my insatiable appetite when it came to sweets. I'm sure her relationship with Stephanie played a little part in her leaving too!

The first month of the year, Celinda began dressing in an androgynous fashion. She cut her very close came out of high heels and started wearing flat masculine shoes. Of course, I made a comment about this new look that could have it been kept to myself. I told her that if I had wanted to be in a relationship with a man, that I would have married one (Bad Randy). In addition, she expressed that I cut out my frequent touches, which initially consisting of tits and ass. Of course, I thought this was a little crazy, so whenever I would touch her, I would touch and feel other parts of her body and follow up with the statement "this is nonsexual touching." The first couple of times, she laughed and joked about our current dilemma. Then I think the little game became annoying to her. The next thing I knew, she was making exit number three. This time she rented a flat from my German friend Martin. Martin and I became friends when I first arrived in Berlin. I answered his aid in the military newspaper seeking friendships with Americans. Of course being naive, I did not realize until we met that he was seeking intimacy. We laughed about the mix up and became friends without the intimacy part. So Celinda, the kids, and I spend lots of time with Martin. Anyway, Martin had fallen in love, and he moved in with his lover. So again, another one of my friends came to her rescue to save her from frustrations of our relationship. We separated after that for a long time. I moved back home on Friday, December 13, 1991, with the kids. Celinda stayed in Berlin and did not return to states until May 1992. I am sure it was because I was filing for divorce and engaged to marry Dr. Denise Davis that November. Well, we know that didn't happen. Once again, I let her back into my heart. OK, now that you know our brief history, let's get back to 1996.

Chapter 10

Jason and I

By mid-July, I was up to forty-five minutes on the stair climber. I'll never forget the evening of July 25, when I was ten minutes into my workout on the stair climber and I felt a drop of sweat on my forehead, and before I reached fifteen minutes, sweat was flowing everywhere. I was filled with jubilation, and tears begin to flow as I increased my pace. Nobody knew that I was crying because my body was drenched with sweat. I never realized how much my profuse sweating that used to annoy and embarrass me would be so missed, needed, and loved. God was making me a new man and giving me a great insight in to what's real.

By exit time number four, I was OK with the absence of cohabiting with Celinda. However, this time it felt different. There was very little communication between us, and she appeared to be angry at me about something and the usual trying to resolve her own personal issues. I knew that this separation situation would become permanent. I physically felt my heart breaking and knew that I would never love this way again. I learned and sang the song "I Can't Make You Love" by Bonnie Rait so much that within a month, Jason had learned the words too and joined me singing periodically.

By the first of August, Jason and I adjusted well with our living conditions reduced by two. Both of us are kind of creatures of habit. We had a ritual in the evenings during the summer. I would be just chilling in the house and Jason would ride his bike out to Green Run High School and play tennis, but would always back in the house before 8:00 p.m. so that we could watch "Moesha." Jason loved Brandy, and Sheryl Ralph made my blood rush! One evening, it was near eight o'clock, and Jason was nowhere in sight. I thought maybe he's running a little late, which I knew was a crazy thought because Jason is always punctual. I thought to leave the house and search for him. Then I thought if something has happen how will they contact me if I am out of the house? I decided to stay by the phone and tried to muster up some happy thoughts. By quarter after eight, I was on borderline of sliding into the crazy mode when the phone rang. I answered the phone, and it was the Sentara Bayside hospital calling telling me that Jason had been admitted. I hung up and in a flash I was there at hospital. I found Jason in one of those stalls in the emergency room stretched out on the bed, awake and smiling. I went over with tears in eyes and gave him a big life hug. The doctor came in and aid that Jason had a seizure. My heart dropped! All that Jason could remember was that he was playing tennis with a guy around my age and next thing he knew he was in an ambulance on his way to the emergency room. I was grateful to people for taking care of my son at Green Run. To this day, I don't know who called 911 or ensured that the ambulance carried all of his personal belongings including his bicycle. Thank you again for I am eternally grateful. The doctor told me that he would let Jason to go home and we needed to make appointment with a neurologist. I asked Jason if he wanted to call his mother and said, "Since I'm being discharged in a few, let's call Mom when we get home." I called Celinda as soon as we arrived home, and she came over immediately and spent the night. I made an appointment to see Dr. Patel at 10:00 a.m. Celinda was in the boys' bathroom getting cleaned up and I was downstairs preparing breakfast when I heard her scream. I ran upstairs only to witness Celinda holding Jason's head in her lap while his body was shaking rapidly. What probably was not much more than a minute seemed like an eternity as I rushed to the phone and called 911. Once Jason's seizure was over, I set him on the bed with arms around him, and we were both crying. I remember saying, "Oh, God, please don't take my son away from me." We just kind of sat there, and Celinda for a minute or so watch us grieve, and then she went downstairs and let in the emergency technicians. They checked Jason out thoroughly and said that there was no need to take him to the emergency room because we had an appointment already scheduled to see Dr. Patel at 10:00 a.m.

We went to see Dr. Patel that morning, and he immediately referred to a neurologist. He prescribed the drug Depicolt, which Jason took for two years and did not experience any more seizures. Celinda for some reason did not like the neurologist; she felt like he's being judgmental, questioning her motherhood. I thought Jason was having the seizures because he stayed intact through cancer, separation, and family drama. He didn't express much about the family's dilemmas, whereas Lamarr truly acted out of his feeling and emotions. The doctor probably did not want to add salt to injury, so he assured us that our current state of affair was not culprit. Once we got back home, I felt tension between the three of us. Then I experienced my first emotion-filled episode with Jason for he made a good point that I was so wrapped up in getting through those radiation treatments five times a week that his feeling were totally overlooked. He stated that no one asked how he felt about watching me reduce to nothing slowly from daily drives from the cancer center. He said that it was not an easy task but rose to the occasion. Then Celinda expressed at a later date how angry she was with me because I did not call her from the hospital instead of waiting until we arrived home. I told her I was not thinking about her at that time, and I let Jason make that decision. I know now that was not an acceptable answer.

The first of August, my siblings/spouses and I met at Mama B's house for a family meeting. Mama B had been complaining about Daddy's worsening Alzheimer's disease and how difficult it was for her take care of him. We started to discuss alternatives when my brother Henry started whining about his upcoming court date. In the mist of his despair, Barbara Sue bluntly stated, "Henry I don't see why you are over there wining about your situation look at what Randy is going through?" Then out of blue, Daddy stated, "What's Randy going through?" At that moment, even though I knew that Daddy was forgetting things, it felt like someone had stuck a knife in my heart and turned it a few times. I did everything in my power to hold back the tears, as Barbara Sue went on and said, "God Daddy, he's dealing with cancer, going through divorce, and Jason just a month ago fell out and had a couple of seizures." There was a moment of silence before lines of communication commenced. Everyone in room made a brief second of eye contact with me and felt their remorse. That is when I discovered that even when you're feeling are at your lowest, people you love can take you even lower.

The result of the big meeting was that the eight of us would take care of our father. He would come and live with Jason and I. Henry and Barbara Sue were responsible for finding him a home nurse. I would change my family room into a bedroom for Daddy, so that he would not have to climb the stairs too often. Within a couple of days, they found a nurse who was eager to take on the challenge of caring for Daddy during the day. That's when they broke the news to Mama B requesting she turn over Daddy's retirement checks so that we could pay the nurse. Mama B was not happy about it; she thought that she got to keep Daddy's money while we cared from him and foot the expense. So within a week's time, another family meeting was scheduled.

We assembled at Mama B's only to find Daddy sitting on their orange couch in tears saying "don't take me from Bee." We were all very emotional at that point, and all the plans that were made instantly went down the drain. From that moment, everything was in Mama B's hands for she was his wife and had the final say so. I left feeling that somehow Daddy would have a bright future, and it was his retirement check that was responsible for the change of heart. It worked out for the best. I was not sure if Jason and I really were ready to take on that responsibility while trying to adjust to the absence of Celinda and Lamarr.

Mid-August 1996 was hernia surgery time. It was an outpatient surgery, so I was happy that I would not have to spend a night in the hospital. I had the honor of Dr. Rahman once more to make the physical invasion and to patch me up. He performed laparoscopic surgery, which started with making a couple of incisions just below my navel for entry of the medical equipment. Once inside, he placed a mesh-like material on the thorn intestinal wall. He stitched me up, which added two beauty marks to an already great work of art. The surgery went great and even waking up from the anesthesia was drama-less. The only problem was the size of my scrotums. I could not believe how large they were; they looked like elephant gonads. I know Winky was not happy with the small image he was projecting laying among the mass of two gigantic nuts.

They say to get over a woman you need to get a different woman. Heeding that advice in August 1996, I mastered using the Internet, frequently visiting the Black Voices Hamptons Roads chat room in hopes of finding a nice lady. I started communicating with a lady that lives in Portsmouth, Virginia, whom I will call Ms. P. Our phone conversations were very stimulating, so we decided to meet one another in person. We gave each other a brief description of ourselves and selected the Ferry dock at Waterside in Norfolk for the physical evaluation. Ms. P rode the Ferry from Portside and arrived at the docks only to find a guy that matched his description. She possessed a few of the physical characteristics, and she looked like she did not put much effort into her appearance. She said, "Oh my god, you really look nice, please forgive me for not fixing myself up." She said that when she met a guy in the past from the Internet, they never matched their description and thought that this date would be a repeat. So I looked over her appearance and walked around Waterside. Then she said that she had never done this before and invited me to her home. I thought what the hell, what do have to lose. She really wasn't that bad. We went to my car in the parking garage and took the Portsmouth tunnel to Portside, where she picked up her automobile and I followed her to her house. She had a nice clean place, which was a go sign being real and all about things like that. We exchanged flirtatious conversation, and just when I thought the moment was right to take things to another level, she said, "I need to tell you something. Please don't be angry but I smoke cigarettes." My facial expression change in a flash and thought to myself this bitch lied to me. All of the lust emptied out of my soul and limited verbal exchanges. I left the premises never to return.

After the Internet disaster, I joined a match-making service located off of Lynnhaven Parkway, across from Lynnhaven Mall. I was required to attend a mandatory interview, take the Myers-Briggs personality assessment, complete a questionnaire of desired qualities in a mate, and be photographed. For $1,000, they would give you six matches and pretty much claimed that I would find the one. Well, maybe it was too soon to embark on such an expensive venture, but the hand gland combat was getting old. I managed to meet three lovely ladies before I became extremely frustrated and stopped using the service.

Lady number one and I shared several stimulating conversation on the telephone. She had a nice voice, and we enjoyed some of the same things. She expressed how she workout and was serious about having and maintaining good health. We arranged for a face-to-face meeting at Apple Bee's on Indian River Road down the street from Tallwood High School. I arrived early and waited patiently to this nice voice. We told each what we would be wearing for identification purposes. A couple of my students were working at Apple Bee's part time, so when I arrived, I received a warm welcome. Lady number one entered the waiting area with a smile and asked if I were Randy. I was immediately focused on her physical appearance. There she was, a high yellow, big hair, butter ball looking at me with eyes of approval. Oh my god, I thought she was replica on my first wicked stepmother Mrs. Alice. I thought how could the match-making service do a thing like this? Did they read my questionnaire? What do they not understand about wanting brown to preferably dark skinned and slim to medium in statue for a candidate? What a downer! I said to myself suck up my friend and go with the flow, you don't have to marry this gal. I had a wonderful time with lady number one that evening over dinner. Unfortunately, I could not get Mrs. Alice out of my head. I just could not see myself waking up to her every morning or any morning as far as I'm concerned. I did not call her anymore and expressed my concerns with the match-making service representative handling my account.

I met lady number two at Apple Bee's also. Now she was a looker. She had a gorgeous face, a beautiful brown skin, a radiant smile, long shapely legs, and a fantastic booty to complete the package. She was divorced with two young children and worked as a nurse. We had a good time so I invited her to the Annual Lawrence Day picnic. My siblings and I would split cost of this grand event that would take place on Labor Day weekend at the Munden Point Park. We always invited our extended family members, friends, and folks from our home church Little Piney Grove Baptist. It was quite a day of fun and games. We had activities for everyone, which included, baseball, basketball, volleyball, horse shoes, bingo (with prizes), and playground equipment for the small kids. The food consisted of hamburgers, hotdogs, bake beans, potato salad, cold slaw, fried chicken, soft drinks, and pastries, and we always had a roasted pig. Anyway, Lady number two came and brought her kids. Most of the men were captivate by her beauty and charm. I guess I was not in the right place mentally for that was our last date. I think the both us were not feeling any chemistry.

Lady number three, lived in Richmond, so Gay gave me that Tuesday in October off to meet this woman. I drove the Impala SS up there to meet her at her home. Lady number three greeted me at the door, and she was definitely easy on the eyes. She was a few years older than me; however, her body was tight and quite appealing. She also had a cockeye, which I found very sexy. You know how Diana Ross's eye sometimes goes off? Well, that's a real turn on for me because I always wondered what is the eye looking at, and since you don't know, you can always fantasize. She had never been married, but she did have a grown gay son. We spent the day walking, talking, and site seeing with each moment together manufacturing chemistry between us. It was late, and I was sitting next to her on the sofa exchanging tongues when I felt Winky rising to the occasion. She indicated that I was more than welcome to join her upstairs, but I turned chicken and opted to start my journey back to Virginia Beach for I had to be at work the next day. We made a date for her to come and spend the weekend in Virginia Beach. Early Friday evening, she arrived right on time. I introduced her to Jason and helped her carry her things to the guest room. On Saturday, we attended a party at my niece Ronnell and her husband Larry's home in Norfolk. I think it was Gino or CeCe's birthday. Lady number three drew favorable comments from the family. On Saturday night, she slipped into my room and engaged in a little extracurricular activity. It was definitely a time of exploring each other's anatomy. She tried all kinds of tricks, but Winky wouldn't cooperate. So after numerous attempts, she finally gave up and we went to sleep. The next day, she returned to Richmond. Then Jason asked, "Hey dad young people must be different from older people. You meet someone one day and sleep with them the next?" I really did not have a good response to that question at that time, so I left well enough alone. Then Jason said that I was portraying the characteristics of a hoe! I was still caught up in my own desires and put those observations from Jason on the back burner.

Lady number three and I made another date. This time, I drove the 54 up to Richmond on a cold Friday to spend the weekend with her. She greeted me with open arms and led me to her bedroom to put my things down. Once there, we jumped on the bed fully dressed and pressed our bodies together. Winky immediately stood up at attention while we were reuniting our lips. She had a dinner reservation for us so we had to put the passion on hold. She drove us to a very nice restaurant in Richmond. We went in and they seated us in a nice romantic spot. We ordered dinner and conversation began. Things were going good, until she called me corny. Then she proceeded to say that she was not used to going out with someone like me. I ask what she meant by that, and she said, "Oh, I am used to going out with macho guys." I felt a deep plug into my heart and did everything in the world to hold back the tears. She made several attempts to clarify her statement. I faked it and said I did not take offense to what she uttered. I asked God not to let me cry at this table and end this dinner date rapidly. He answered my prayer and before I knew it, we were back at her house. I ran upstairs to gather my things and head for door. She grabbed me and said I did hurt your feeling didn't I? I agreed and rapidly ran to the street and jumped in the 54, only to have her in her I-don't-want-to-start mode. I prayed, Oh Lord, please don't let me be stuck here with this woman. Finally, the 54 started and I was on interstate 64 in flash. That was one cold ride home. The window on the driver's side of the 54 would not completely go up. So my face and upper body was freezing while the heat blowing from below was burning up my feet. Lady number three called several times and sent me a letter to patch up things. However, I had shared my illnesses and body parts (those that worked anyway) with her only to receive ridicule did not set well with my psychological state of being. I decided after that de-masculinizing experience that match-making service was not something I that wanted to explore any further.

At end of February 1997, Frances said that she has a girlfriend that she wanted me to meet and felt like we would hit it off. I took Frances's girlfriend's phone number and gave her a call. She had a raspy, whiny voice and over conversation on the phone lacked substance. I thought to myself, her voice has nothing to do with it since I had been down the road hearing nice voices and finding the opposite upon the physical meeting. We scheduled a time to meet at Bally's one evening during the middle of the week. There I was waiting in the parking lot at Bally's when this grey Toyota pulls up and parks next to the 54. What a beautiful face, an inviting smile, and eyes of lust, and her head cocked to the side as she pulled into the parking spot and stopped. I could feel my blood rushing. Out stepped a dark chocolate, sexy, lean, long-legged, hot mama with large poppy brown eyes. Oh yea, I was feeling this chick and said to myself, Frances you have done good! We bantered around each other like dogs in heat exchanging small talk. Then DC said she needed to pick up a card for a friend and invited me to ride with her to the card shop. I quickly accepted and when I got into her car, it was stick shift. Oh yea, I was definitely getting into DC. The chemistry between us (call it lust if want) continued to intensify with every moment together. I wanted to make love to her that evening; however, there was Jason's voice in the back of head. So we made a date for the weekend, which worked out well because Jason was spending the day with Celinda on Saturday in Hampton. DC came over on Saturday, and it wasn't long before intimacy filled the den. I had not had intercourse since December 1995, so I had was filled with immense anxiety about satisfying her sexy desires. Well, Winky was working so we went to work. It wasn't

long before the explosive ejection and my breathing was so intense that
DC thought I was having a heart attack. After a couple of minutes, my
breathing returned to normal, and I explained to her about the scar tissue
in my chest from the radiation treatment.

DC and I started going out at least twice week. DC even went bike
riding with me to the oceanfront one Saturday. What a gal! In addition, she
met all of my siblings, their families, went down to my home church, and
met many of my extended family members. I was definitely feeling DC;
however, I made sure whenever we did "the do," Jason was not at home or
we copulated at DC's apartment. By mid-May, Jason was going to Orlando,
Florida, for an annual band competition with Tallwood's band. I thought
that this would be a go time for DC and I to experience cohabitation
during Jason's absence. I gave her a key, and she came over the evening
Jason left the city. We had a good time and felt that maybe things are going
to work between us. Jason's bus was due to return to Tallwood at 11:00
a.m. on Sunday. I told DC that I would leave early and wait until Jason's
bus arrived. However, when I arrived at Tallwood, one of parents said that
the band instructor called and said that the bus would be two hours late.
So I drove back home and just I was approaching the house from Lake
Tahoe Street, I spotted DC at back door smoking a cigarette. I turned left
on Seven Springs Court, pulled in the driveway, and rushed into the house.
I met DC in the pantry off the kitchen where she had just closed the back
door. She asked Jason's whereabouts. I gave the details and then asked her
if she had been smoking. She looked me dead in the eyes and said "No, I
have not been smoking, I don't smoke." I thought this bitch just lied to me.
Well, you know what happened after that? At that moment, I decided to
kiss dating good-bye and focus on being there for Jason for the remainder
of time that he lived with me while in high school. He was junior then, so
I only had another year to conquer this commitment. I held true to this
commitment for I did not date again until Jason graduated from Tallwood
and went out of state to college. It's a good thing that in my early twenties I
read and mastered the techniques from the book *101 Ways of Masturbation*.
Believe me when I say those skills certainty came in handy during my
period of abstinence.

Chapter 11

Lamarr Completes
Basic Training and Surprise

Lamarr completed basic training and Celinda moved to an apartment in Hampton. So we all planned to attend his graduation. I purchased a Rodeo for Lamarr that he would be responsible for making $450 a month car payments. Celinda, Rosemary (one of Celinda's closest girlfriends), Jason, and I loaded up the Rodeo and headed Interstate 95 South for South Carolina. There was a little tension in on the way; however, it was tolerable. Whenever I drove, Jason sat in the front seat, and when Celinda drove, Rosemary sat up front. Celinda was pulled over by the state trooper for speeding. She got quite agitated when the state trooper let another car driven by a light-skinned woman continue on her journey without a ticket. She even questioned the state trooper of his unfair actions. He responded, "I did not pull that car over." He then wrote Celinda a ticket. Jason and I just looked at each other and kept silent, whereas Celinda and Rosemary banter back and forth about that unpleasant encounter. We arrived the day before the graduation ceremony, so we got a room at a local hotel. Once Jason and I got settled in the room, we went across the street to Burger King. I must say that was the best-tasting whopper that I have ever put in my mouth. The burger was grilled to perfection, and the lettuce, tomatoes, and onions tasted like they were just harvested.

The next day, the graduation was beautiful and I saw a tremendous amount of accomplishment in Lamarr's eyes. He made my heart smile. Then we made him smile when I threw him the keys to his new Black

Rodeo while looking for the Impala SS. I informed him that I purchased the vehicle on credit and that he would be responsible for making the $450 car payment plus the auto insurance. He was so happy and said that it would not be problem. At that moment, I was disappointed in myself for not being able just to give it to him without a car note. Oh well, maybe in another life. The trip back was not so bad. I remember some conversation exchanged between Celinda and I, but nothing to brag about.

By November of that year, I had exhausted all creative measures to cover the monthly expenses. All of the credit cards were maxed out, totaling $94,182.78 of debt. Attorney Koch had encouraged me to file a chapter 7 bankruptcy a few months back. I just could not do it then for I had been so anal in the past about meeting my financial obligations. I had never been late on any payment in my life. Unfortunately, my financial state was killing me inside, so I finally agreed to follow his advice. He instructed me to continue to pay the mortgage and the household bills but don't send another dime to my creditors. He said when the credits start calling, just let them know you have filed for bankruptcy and give them my number.

Thanksgiving and Christmas carried true to its tradition, just Celinda less. My interaction with Celinda was slim to none. During the holidays, she stopped by a couple of times to see the boys. One evening, she came over wearing a form-fitting dress and four-inch pumps, and when I opened the door to let her in, my all-time low sexual desires spiked. Once I greeted her, I immediately ran upstairs and relieved Winky of his frustration.

Barbara Sue hosted Thanksgiving that year in Baltimore, Maryland. The food was great, and fellowship was wonderful. The big excitement though Frances car was off the street just a few feet from Barbara Sue's home. This was the third time this same car had been stolen.

Christmas was at Olivia and Ronald's house, and again we feasted and just enjoyed the fellowship. Below is the Christmas card I sent that year.

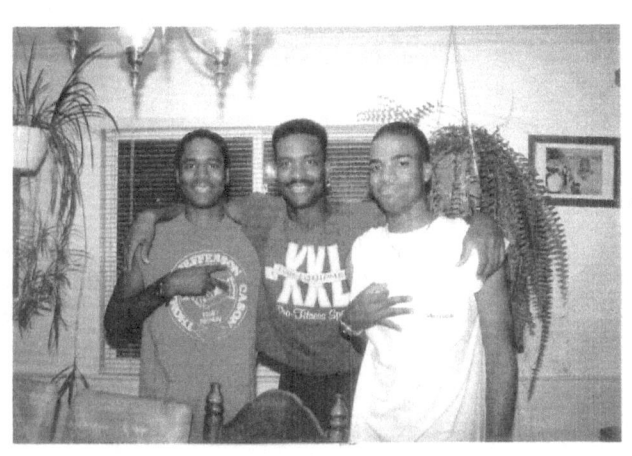

Why the? smiles? It's been a year of Challenges!

Merry Christmas and Happy New Year from the Lawrence's. Randy, Lamonr & Jason

Why the muscles? God gave us the strength to endure these Challenges!

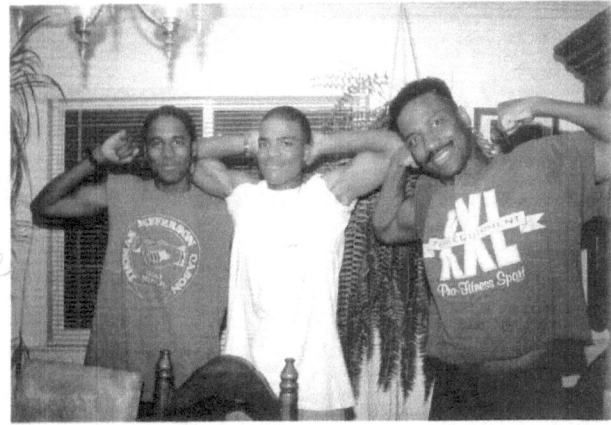

In December 1996, I followed Attorney Koch instructions and did not pay one creditor. In January 1997, the creditors started ringing my phone of the hook. Once I gave them Attorney Koch's number, by the end of February 1997, the calls ceased. What burden lifted, and I thank the Lord for giving me such a caring and outstanding attorney. However, filing for the big "B" haunted my financial self-esteem. How could I have let myself get into this predicament? It was just another factor in my life making me more humble than I already was.

The year 1997 revealed very little communication with Celinda. Celinda was working on getting us a divorce; she said that her lawyer would do it for $500. So I took the back seat and started to wait patiently for the big "D" to strike. In February 1997, Lamarr called me from his Military Occupation Training School in Paris Island, South Carolina, to give me the news that his girlfriend, who according to him looked just like Jada Pinkett, named Kia Hicks, was pregnant and the baby was due in October. I congratulated him, and as time went on, I became more and more excited about the birth of my first grandchild.

In January 1997, we found that Daddy was in the early stages of Alzheimer's disease. This was an inception of a family meeting to see how we care for my father. All of my siblings, their spouses, and Mama B would sit in on these meetings. I had no idea what the future would bring. I do know the eight of us loved and respected Daddy. He was the provider. Bear with me as I take you back in time. It was September 22, 1957, and what a day! It was my parents' wedding anniversary, mama's birthday, and my birthday. Mama prepared a gustatory birthday cake, with four blue candles while waiting for Daddy to return with her wonderful surprise. Suddenly, Mama was stricken with excruciating pains in her abdominal area. She was taken to bed and Great Mama Diszer arrived to administer first aid. Daddy soon returned home and immediately rushed Mama to DePaul Hospital, in Norfolk, for the Virginia Beach Hospital would not serve black people. It was too late when they arrived at De Paul. Mama started to hemorrhage and died shortly after being admitted. After Mama's dolorous departure, Daddy got all of kids back together and raised us to adulthood. He was definitely the provider who cared for the eight of us through thick and thin.

In July 1997, between Jason's junior and senior year, he was accepted to a Summer Engineering Program and the University of Vermont. I made a timeshare exchange for a place in New Hampshire up in the White Mountains. Early Sunday morning, Jason and I drove the Impala SS up to Vermont, and once we arrived at the university, I made sure he got settled for this three-day summer program. I then proceeded to New Hampshire for my first solo vacation in a place where I did not know anyone. It was a great experience. I discovered that I could have fun without company and that was edifying in itself. On that Wednesday, I went back to the University of Vermont to attend the program's closing ceremony. I got to see the projects that Jason worked on while he was there. After the awards were presented, Jason packed up and we went back to the White Mountains. I'm sure the most exciting thing that Jason would be able to remember about his stay in the White Mountains was when we went horseback riding.

Then in the end of July 1997, Celinda agreed to meet at a neutral place to make a car switch. Even though she was still making the car payments on Impala SS, Jason and I had the car for that year while she drove the Grand Am since it was better on gas. We met at a gas station in Norfolk. When we got out of our cars to make the exchange, our eyes met, and I started to burn with passion just viewing her sexy body and seeing that come-jump-my-bones look in her eyes. My physical attraction was so intense when we exchanged car keys that Winky emerged into a huge erection. The chemistry between us was so thick you can't cut it with a knife. I took the keys from her hot hands and immediately jumped into the Grand Am to avoid making a fool out myself from a lack of self-control. We looked at each as we drove off the parking lot, and I began deep breathing to slow down my heartbeat.

On August 1, 1997, Mattie and Olivia gave Kia a baby shower at my house. Kia's mother, Diana Hicks, came down for a couple of days and stayed with me so that she could attend the baby shower. Celinda and I both took her out on separate occasions to open the lines of communication between us. The day of the baby shower, Lamarr, Jason, and I were the only males present. My sister as always had a party filled with events that kept the ladies laughing and thinking/moving around. I was thinking how blessed I was to be born in such a loving/caring family who had been an imponderable support system. Lamarr and Kia were so pleased at the turn out and all of wonderful gifts that they received.

By mid-August, Jason, Olivia, Deedee, and I traveled to Massanutten for a week of vacation in the mountains. During the middle of our vacation, I had to travel back home to attend my bankruptcy hearing. Again, Attorney Koch came to my rescue. I had to say very little, and he handled everything. God I love that man. All of the debt was flushed, including the $23,129.75 that Lamarr still owed on his Rodeo, which had been repossessed months ago. I was moving a little faster, and a tremendous weight was lifted from my shoulders. By mid-October, my discharge of debt from bankruptcy documents arrived. I was in a small state of shock; $117,312.53 of debt gone, and a new beginning financially for me. I still got to keep my house, cars, and both timeshares.

Ain't God good! On October 23, 1997, Kia gave birth to our first grandson, whom she named Cortne Taylor Lawrence. The Grand Pum Pom came into our lives and what a blessing he has been. Lamarr came home before the event to pick up the video camera to film the birth of his son. However, Kia ended having a C-section so Lamarr did not do any recording of the tremendous event. Cortne's arrival increased the communication between Celinda and I from the joy shared from the entrance of this little man into our lives. And of course, Lamarr was strutting around like a proud peacock. I was just so elated and dying to hold the little man in my arms. I created another Christmas letter and mailed it out to family and friends.

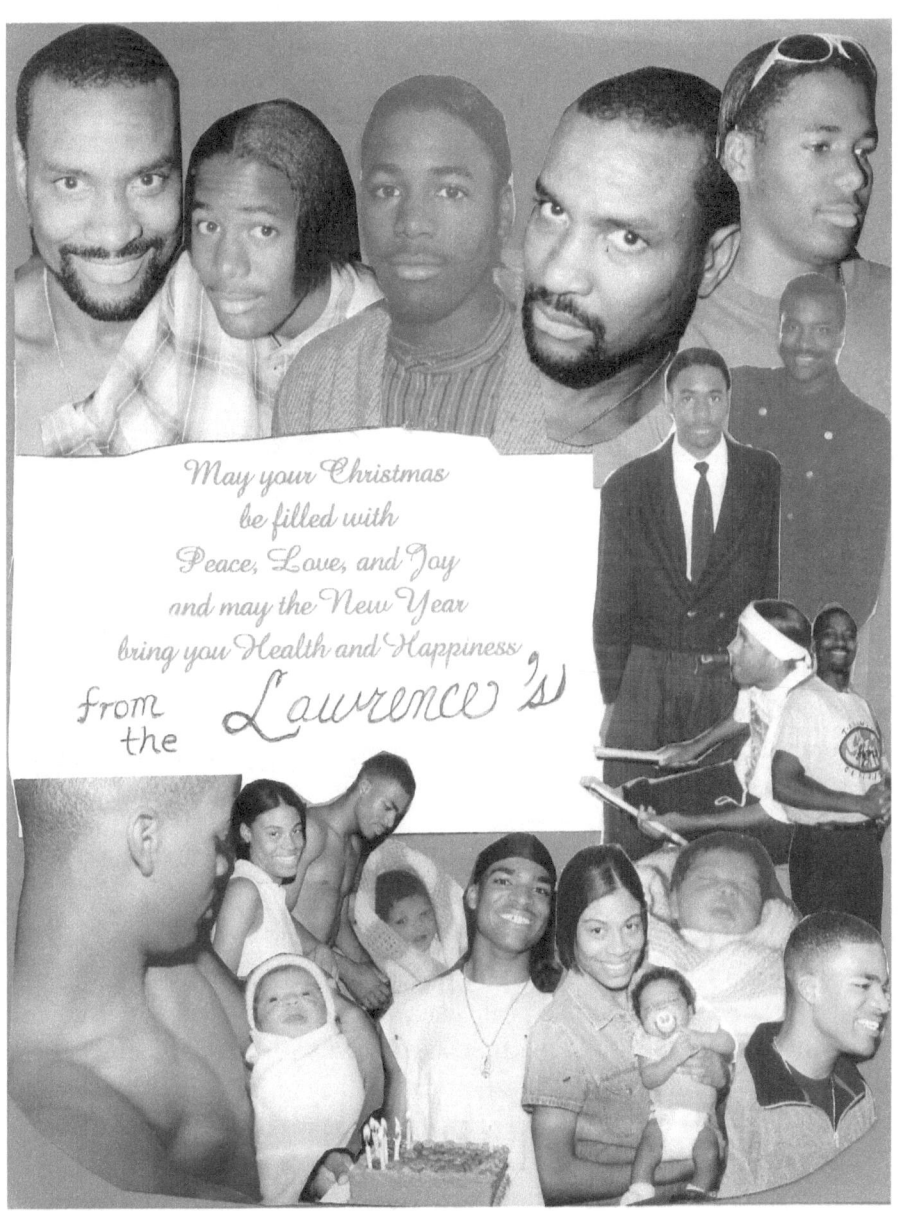

May your Christmas
be filled with
Peace, Love, and Joy
and may the New Year
bring you Health and Happiness

from the Lawrence's

In Christmas 1997, Lamarr came home. I suspected that he was using drugs, so I asked him, and of course he denied using any illegal substances. I let it ride and stored my suspicions in the back of my mind. We did the usual ritual of opening our gifts and taking pictures. I made pancakes and bacon, and we ate while recapping old memories. We had the usual dinner at Olivia and Ronald, which is again great. We reaped the benefits of food, fun, and fellowship. Jackie was visiting home from Puerto Rico, so we hooked up a couple of days after Christmas for a road trip. We drove the Grand Am over 2,000 miles to Miami, Florida, and back to Virginia Beach with a few stops along the way. We left on Monday, December 30, and drove 1,000 miles straight to Miami with a few pit stops. We arrived in Bal Harbor, and Deborah welcomed us with open arms. Deborah had a great schedule of events planned for our stay. She took us down to South Beach, to Parade in Miami, and out to dinner a couple of nights. We got a chance to meet Steve, her new beau. On New Year's Eve, Deborah, her friend name Michael (whom she nicknamed Tyrone because she always had to reach down in her purse and pay his way wherever they went), Jack, and I attended an Alcoholic Anonymous party. There was a five-dollar cover charge, and when we arrived at the entrance, Tyrone said, "Oh my goodness, forgot and left my wallet at home," so there was Deborah reaching down in her purse one more time. We had a great time and danced like crazy. Deborah said she had a lady that she wanted me to meet. I always told Deborah that I wanted a black Deborah Jones. So Deborah wanted me to meet this black lady named Deborah Jones. We met and she was nice and all. I just had a hard time getting past the gold tooth. The day after New Year's, we started our journey back to Virginia Beach, making a couple of stops along the way. Our first stop was in Paris Island, South Carolina, to Kia's apartment. There I got chance to see and hold my grandson for the first time—Cortne Taylor Lawrence, what a grandchild to hold. Even then I knew that he had a gentle spirit. Jackie took turns holding Cortne and snapping photographs of each other. We visited with Kia and baby Cortne for about one hour and a half and hit the road again to visit one of Jackie's old boyfriend named Grant. It was my first time meeting this guy that Jack had spoken about with butterflies. We arrived there pretty late, so after the informal introduction and about an hour of communication, we when went to bed. The next morning, Grant joined Jack and me at the I Hop for breakfast. We said our good-byes at the I Hop, and Jackie and I were on the road again. Our last stop was at the South of the Board for a delicious meal before arriving back in Virginia later that evening.

Chapter 12

The Divorce in 1998

In January 1998, I received a phone call from Lamarr stating that he had come up positive on a urinal analysis and there may be a chance that he would be kicked out of the Marine Corps. Shortly after that conversation, Henry called and asked me if I could video his presentation at one of the local churches, and I agreed. I pulled out the video camera that Lamarr returned before Thanksgiving, and there was still a tape in the cam recorder. I took the videotape and inserted it into the VCR to find a blank space where I could start the new recording. When the imagines appeared on the screen, there was neither Cortne nor Kia, but the imagines consisted of several young men circulating, taking a hit off a joint taking. When I stepped closer trying make out the imagines, I could not believe my eyes when one of the faces was Lamarr, with him actually taking a hit. Well, needless to say, I could have confirmed my suspicions months before if I had only watched that tape Lamarr left in the camera back in November.

In February 1998, after numerous Lawrence family meeting, it was a unanimous decision that the sons would take a night to sit with Daddy and help him to bed. Mama B said that it was just too much for her handle anymore. I chose Tuesday evening. It was so hard watching Daddy loose his memory and revert back to childhood. After I had a few emotional breakdowns caring for Daddy, I made up my mind that I would not get caught up in sympathy but just go with moment. Here are a few stories that I would like to share at Mama B's with Daddy. The first evening I sat with Daddy, he was watching television in the family room while I was working on some work from school at the kitchen table. Daddy turned and asked, "Hey Randy, can I stay up until 9 o'clock? I want to finish this show on TV." His bed time was usually at 8:30 p.m. Of course I responded with sure Daddy. That's when I realized that our roles were beginning to reverse. The nights that I would care for Daddy, I would always tell him it's 8 o'clock Daddy, it's time to get ready for bed. He would go into his bedroom and put on his pajama. Once he was dressed for bed, he would then call for me and I would help him in on the right of the bed closest to the window. Then I asked if he was comfortable with his position in the bed, if not I'll move him to the position he desired. Daddy was not a little man, so whenever I started to move him physically, the scar tissue would shift in my chest and I would start to gasp for air. This was nothing serious. It always happens when I attempted something new my body was not used to, which stem from the radiation treatments in 1995/1996. Then, I tucked him in and say good night and turned off the lights and leave the room.

One evening, Daddy was getting ready for bed. He called for me, but this time it was for help. Once I got in the bedroom, Daddy was sitting on the edge of bed frustrated shaking his head because he could not get his pants off. He said, "Randy I don't know what's wrong, I can't get my pants off." I said let's have look Daddy. Oh, I see you forgot to take your shoes off first. He said in excitement, "Oh, is that the problem?" We shared a laugh, and I helped him with his shoes and the pants, and we completed the nightly ritual.

One evening, Patsy substituted for me because I had a commitment at school. When I arrived home that evening, I received a call from Patsy explaining her evening with Daddy. She said, "What have you done to Daddy?" When I was helping him to get to bed, he would not sit or get in. I said to him what's wrong Daddy? He stated that Randy always let me get in the bed on the right side. So we went to the right side and got into the bed. Then he started taking deep breathes like he was upset. I said what's wrong Daddy. He responded with Randy always straightens me up in the bed. So I straightened him out in the bed. I got ready to turn off the light and the breathing started again. I asked what is wrong now Daddy? He responds Randy always tucks me in." Patsy and I laughed so much that evening.

With lines of communication established somewhat between Celinda and I, I inquired about the status of the divorce proceeding. She said that she was having problems coming with the $500. I contacted Attorney

Koch, and of course he came to my rescue once again. He said he could do the divorce for $185. I told Celinda that I would pay for the divorce and she could save herself $500. Attorney Koch immediately got the ball rolling and before I knew it, the date was set for Celinda, me, and a witness to sign the documents parting us legally. The day of our appointment, Olivia came with me as witness, and of course Celinda was a no show. A young lawyer was handling the proceeding. He said that it was OK that Celinda did not show because there were other means of obtaining her signatures of the documents. Olivia was all up in the young lawyer's business. I'll tell you that when we left his office, Olivia could probably tell you the young man's underwear size.

In March 1998, I called Celinda to see if the three of us could celebrate Jason's eighteenth birthday together. She agreed, and we decided that we would pick her up and go to a restaurant at Hampton. So on March 29, 1998, Jason and I headed to Hampton in the 54 Chevy for his eighteenth birthday celebration. Once we went through the Hampton Road tunnel, I noticed that Jason did not take the exit to go to Celinda's apartment complex. I remained silent. I thought that maybe Jason knew a different route. I had Celinda's home address but had never been to her apartment. Jason pulled up in a driveway of a white house with blue shutters. I said Jason does your mother live here? He said, "Oh yea, Dad, didn't you know that Mom brought a house?" I responded with I do now. Celinda came out on the porch looking good enough to eat with a grand smile. As we got out of the 54 and approached the house, I notice an automobile parked on the street right in front of her house. Celinda stated, "I hope you don't mind I have prepared a meal here, so I thought that we could eat here instead of eating out." I was OK with that suggestion, so we entered her home. I congratulated her on purchasing a home, and she offered to show me around her place. I agreed, and the tour began. We viewed inside out except the master bedroom. Once the tour was done, I made a mental note, no master bedroom tour and a car parked on the curve in the front of house. Oh yea, I thought, huh hum she has got a nigger up in here. Celinda went to the kitchen to work on the meal and made small talk with me while I was standing in dining room. Then all of sudden, a man came out of the master bedroom. Jason looked at me in shock. Celinda immediately said, "Hey Randy this is a friend of mine, Will, he just stopped over for a few minutes; however, he will not be staying." I extended my hand and walked up to Will, shook his hand, and expressed that it was nice meeting him.

We still had a few minutes before the meal, so Celinda suggested that Jason give us a selection on his electric keyboard. Jason's playing left a lot to be desired for he was so nervous and shook up about Will's presence. Shortly after Jason finished his selection, Will left. Then Celinda, Jason, and I sat down for a very tasty meal. After the meal, we drove out the park and hiked a nature trail and then we brought Celinda back to her house.

Once we were on road, Jason turned to me and said, "Dad, I am so sorry; I did not know Mom's boyfriend was going to be there." I said to him, Jason it's a good thing that I am over your mother. However, that was a pretty dirty thing for her to do. Then Jason said, "Well Dad, you have had some girlfriends." I said yes this is true; however, I have never invited your mother to our house and parade a woman out of my bedroom. It was pretty much silence the rest of the way home.

The next evening, Celinda called to apologize about Will being at her place. She stated he stopped by that morning to use the bathroom. I thought to myself, that's strange if he had just stopped to use the bathroom, how come he did not use guest bathroom which was located very close to the front door. I told her that I was not bothered at all, in fact I found Will to be a very nice guy. And that I hope Will will be able to make her happy. Then added if I were a woman, I would consider dating him myself. We shared a chuckle. However, I heard in Celinda's voice that the plan to make me jealous failed.

On April 1, 1998, our divorce became legal. I realized then our marriage was over and the divorce made it permanent. As much as I loved and desired Celinda, I knew that the two of us being together would destroy my existence. The cancer cleared my vision and revealed things that I was not willing to accept in the past about my relationship with the lady that I fell in love with at first sight in the library at NSU in 1975. After sharing extreme highs, extreme lows, and no in-betweens with this truly exciting lady, how am I going shake this feeling. How am I going to kill this burning desire to be with her physically? The answer my friend is I have accomplished none of things listed above. I have accepted that I will always love and be attached to Celinda and have learned that some things that are good to you aren't necessarily good for you. With that said, I have embraced Dionne Warwick's song "I Know I'll Never Love This Way Again."

I know you are wondering what made me stay and continue to love this lady, which is depicted as a cold and selfish woman. Remember these were only a few moments in time that I experienced so much grief from her actions. I can truly say that fourteen of twenty years that Celinda and I married was simply off the charts with happiness for me. She was very affectionate, thoughtful, always giving, and forever changing her appearance. During times when she was not depressed, our moments were tender and our conversation always stimulating. We dated so much after we got married, whether it was a hike on a nature trail or attending the opera, it was never a dull moment for me. My brother-in-law Ronald kind of summed up my relationship with Celinda when he said, "Men usually date a woman to get married; however, I got married to have a woman to date." I always felt like a stud when I had her on my arms. Making love to her was more than a physical release; it was a combination of totally ecstasy and a union of two souls messed together usually producing an orgasm that literally started from the tip of my toes. She always respected my caregiver's spirit and tolerated all of ventures of me trying to help others or filling my life during the holidays with new friends when we were in the military to fill the void of not being around my family. She was comfort for me during my low moments of grief, especially when my Mama Sue died in 1985.

Celinda was very creative and possessed stage presence that would keep an audience focused. Over years, she acted in several plays and produced/participated some really good programs throughout my tenure in the Military, and I even helped in a couple of them. I remember the first military dance we attended. I taught Celinda how to do the hustle when we living in that tiny blue and white trailer in Clarksville, Tennessee. The dance was held on Fort Campbell, Kentucky. That night, Celinda was wearing a green uneven layer flowing dress and four-inch pumps. The moment we hit the floor and flowed with the music in unison, I knew instantly that dancing together was just another way to elevate our connection.

Celinda was a very loving and caring mother. The boys simply adore her, along with all of our nieces, nephews, stray kids, and mentally changed adults that I would bring home periodically. She always made them feel at home and never ridicule me for always sharing our family time with others. One good example of her good nature was the summer of 1986 when we stationed at Fort Stewart, Georgia. Living in Hinesville, we kept five additional kids, which consisted of my brother Henry's three kids, Wilbert

Jr., Melissa, and Lee, my sister Patsy's son Chris, and Rosemary's (Celinda's girlfriend) two sons Boo and Jason. It was a great summer for Lamarr and Jason having so many young people living under one roof, and Celinda spent most of the time with them.

Celinda was also the pastry chef from heaven. She could shake and bake simultaneously, which kept me simulated inside out. Once she would complete one of her pastries, she would receive validation on her creation from the expression on my face and portions that I would consume. Jason would always enhance her validation after taking one bite of whatever she prepared and immediately jump up from the table and do a little booty dance. I knew it became hard for her when I became diabetic. However, she started experimenting with sugar pastries. They were good but I just didn't get the buzz that I was accustomed to with real sugar.

Last and certainly not the least, Celinda was my best friend and "Scrabble Buddy." I felt comfortable sharing even my darks secrets with her. She understood my needs and never appeared to be judgmental when I would get a wild hair up my butt. So I was married to someone that I loved inside out and always got charge out of being in her presence. The majority of the time that we spent together was always a happy time for me and was usually filled with laughter. What a void her departure left in my life. I thank God that she was not my main source of joy. "This joy that I have the world didn't give to me. The world didn't give it and the world can't take it away."

Chapter 13

Lessons Learned from Simultaneously Surviving Cancer and Celinda

1. After being stripped of the greatest individual pleasures, my inner peace and joy was definitely from within and a gift from God.
2. My relationship with God was based on more than him giving me good health.
3. People who love you don't want to hear about how bad you feel or how much you are hurting because they really don't want to feel bad or hurt too. I know you have heard the expression when you hurt, I hurt too! No one really wants to hurt.
4. When you are sharing your life with someone you love, it is never reciprocated in an equal volume.
5. You do not have control over anyone with the exception of yourself.
6. When it comes to matters of the heart, the feelings are really controlled by our thoughts.
7. A broken heart is more painful than a broken bone, for the bone heals much faster.
8. Forgiveness is the key to releasing you from turmoil when it involves relationship.
9. It's the right thing to forgive, but for heaven's sake, don't forget or you will have a repeat!
10. If I cannot experience a feeling greater than what I had with Celinda, I'd rather be alone.
11. It is OK to be alone!

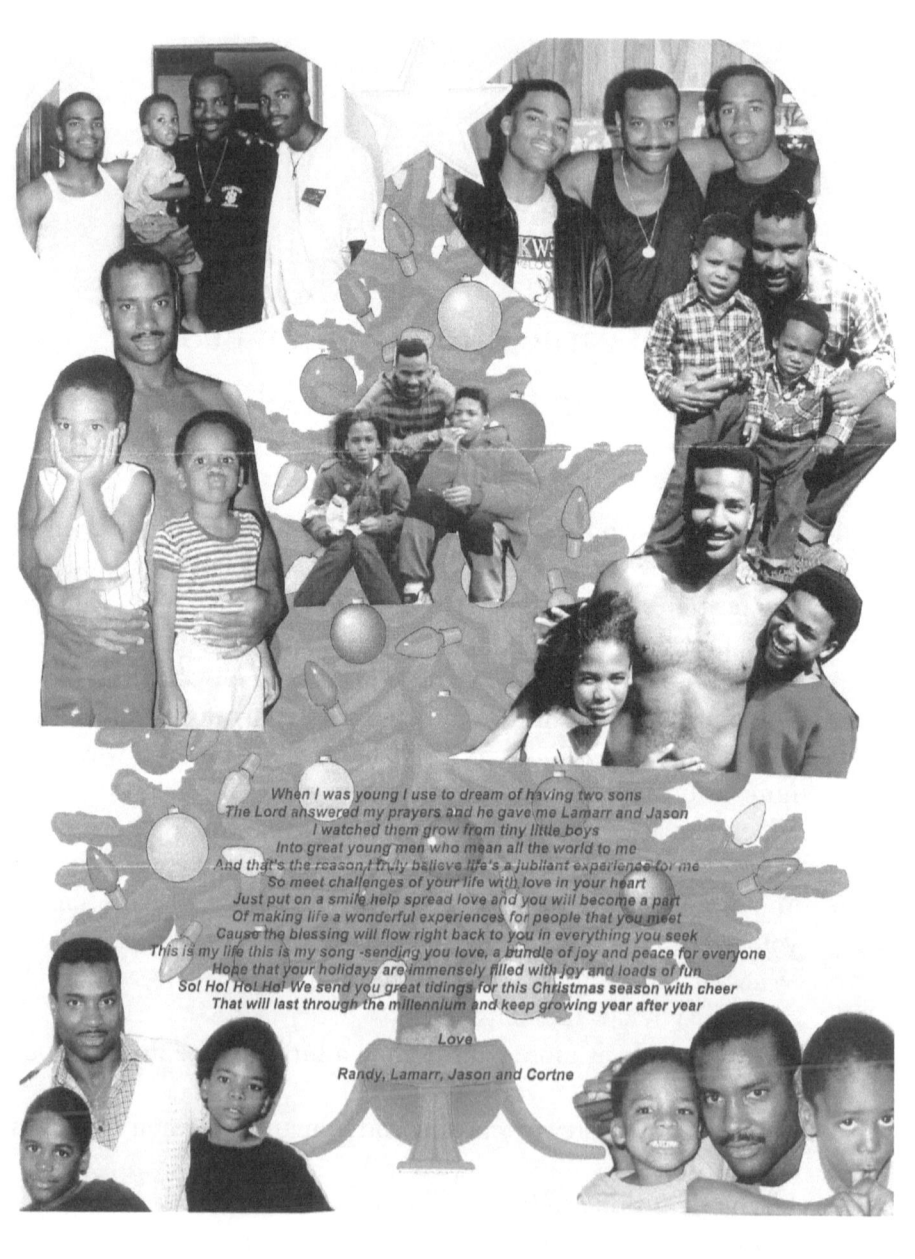

When I was young I use to dream of having two sons
The Lord answered my prayers and he gave me Lamarr and Jason
I watched them grow from tiny little boys
Into great young men who mean all the world to me
And that's the reason I truly believe life's a jubilant experience for me
So meet challenges of your life with love in your heart
Just put on a smile help spread love and you will become a part
Of making life a wonderful experiences for people that you meet
Cause the blessing will flow right back to you in everything you seek
This is my life this is my song -sending you love, a bundle of joy and peace for everyone
Hope that your holidays are immensely filled with joy and loads of fun
So! Ho! Ho! Ho! We send you great tidings for this Christmas season with cheer
That will last through the millennium and keep growing year after year

Love

Randy, Lamarr, Jason and Cortne